Nutrition & Poverty

Nutrition: *A Global View*

Books in This Series

Nutrition & Politics

Nutrition & Poverty

Nutrition & Science

Nutrition & Society

Nutrition & You

Nutrition & Poverty

Rae Simons

AlphaHouse Publishing
New York

Nutrition: A Global View
Nutrition & Poverty

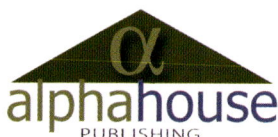

alphahouse
PUBLISHING

AlphaHouse Publishing
A Division of PEMG Publishing Group, Inc.
201 Harding Avenue
Vestal, New York 13850
www.alphahousepublishing.com

First Printing
9 8 7 6 5 4 3 2 1
ISBN: 978-1-934970-30-0
ISBN (set): 978-1-934970-28-7
     Library of Congress Control Number: 2008930656
Author: Simons, Rae

Cover design by Wendy Arakawa.
Interior design by MK Bassett-Harvey.

Printed in India by International Print-O-Pac Limited

An ISO 9001 Company

Contents

Introduction 6

1. What Is Nutrition? 9

2. What Is Poverty? 29

3. Nutrition & Poverty in the Developing World 45

4. Nutrition & Poverty in the Developed World 61

5. What Is the World Doing? 75

For More Information 90

Glossary of Nutrition-Related Terms 93

Bibliography 106

Index 109

Picture Credits 111

About the Author and the Consultant 112

Introduction to Nutrition:

A Global View

Many young adults are used to looking at nutrition in the context of health classes and home economics classes. Most of them know that nutrition is a critical component for healthy development, one that is connected to energy levels, strong bones and teeth, clear skin, reduced risk for infectious diseases, and other physical outcomes. But students may be far less aware that nutrition also has global consequences. It is an issue that pertains to social studies, economics, current events, and science studies.

In our global world, nutrition issues have enormous importance. Food crises and world hunger are only the most visible and urgent tip of the malnourishment iceberg. Beneath the world's waters lurks an even more pervasive danger. At least one-fifth of the worldwide loss of years of life to death and to disability is due to hunger and undernutrition. If diet-related chronic diseases (such as diabetes, obesity, and hypertension) are taken into consideration, some experts believe that as much as one-half of the world's illnesses and mortality can be attributed to malnutrition.

As future citizens and leaders, young adults need to understand that investing in the world's nutrition is vital to the well-being of the global community. Improved nutrition empowers people and communities; it fuels the development process and leads to political, economic, and social renewal. Empowered and well-nourished communities are also less likely to be drawn into wars and violent conflicts. In an increasingly interconnected world, the payoff for global good nutrition is higher than ever.

The United Nations is well aware of this connection; the rights of all individuals to appropriate and adequate nutrition are embedded in six of the universal proclamations included in the 1990 World Declaration and Plan of Action on the Survival, Protection and Development of Children. Kofi Annan, former Secretary General of the United Nations, has written:

> The world knows what is needed to end malnutrition. With a strong foundation of cooperation between local communities, non-governmental organizations, governments, and international agencies, the future—and the lives of our children—can take the shape we want and they deserve, of healthy growth and development, greater productivity, social equity, and peace.

The books in this series, Nutrition: A Global View, will help students build the knowledge base and the perspectives necessary to help achieve these vital goals.

—*Dr. Peter Vash*

Here's what you need to know

- Good nutrition comes from the parts of food that allow our bodies to do their jobs.
- Malnutrition means not getting enough of the foods you need to be healthy.
- The nutrients (the part of food that provides nutrition) that your body needs are calories, carbohydrates, fat, protein, vitamins, minerals, fiber, and water.
- A calorie is a way to measure how much energy a food offers your body.
- You need 1 gram (about a third of an ounce) of protein per kilogram of weight (0.4 grams per pound).
- Carbohydrates give you energy. If you eat too many carbohydrates, they will be converted into body fat.
- About 30 percent of your daily calories should come from fat in order for your body to be healthy.
- You need smaller amounts of vitamins and minerals, but these substances found in foods are still very important to good health.
- Poverty and malnutrition go together.

1 What Is Nutrition?

Nutrition is what we get from the food we eat. It's the part of food that gives our bodies what they need to function—to live and move around, to think and breathe, play and work. Without nutrition, we could not survive for very long.

Malnutrition is when our bodies don't get all the nutrients they need. A person with malnutrition is often more likely to catch diseases. Malnutrition can also affect brain function, eyesight, and the function of various body organs. If a child has malnutrition, she may not grow as tall or weigh as much as would be normal for other children her age. If a pregnant woman is malnourished, the fetus within her may not develop normally.

Nutrients

The food we eat contains different types of nutrients (the materials that supply us with nutrition). These nutrients include calories, carbohydrates, fats, proteins, vitamins, minerals, fiber, and water. We need some of all these; our bodies are healthiest and work their best when they have

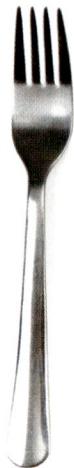

Nutrition Facts

Per 1 meal

Amount	% Daily Value
Calories 0	
Fat 0 g	**0 %**
Carbohydrate 0 g	**0 %**
Protein 0 g	

Not a significant source of saturated fat, trans fat, cholesterol, sodium, fiber, sugars, vitamin A, vitamin C, calcium or iron.

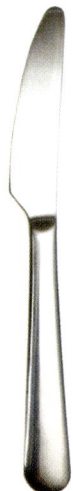

a balanced diet made of different foods that contain all the nutrients.

Most foods contain a mix of some or all of the different kinds of nutrients. Some nutrients are required every day (or nearly every day), while others aren't needed as often. Scientists sometimes sort nutrients into two categories: the macronutrients—the ones we need in large quantities, including carbohydrates, fat, fiber, protein, and water—and the micronutrients—the ones we don't need as much of, such as vitamins and minerals. Poor health can be caused by an imbalance of nutrients, whether an **excess** or a **deficiency**.

The macronutrients (except for fiber and water) provide our bodies with energy. They are the body's fuel, and they contain calories. Vitamins and minerals do not give us energy, but our bodies need them for other reasons.

Calories

If you live in one of the world's **developed** countries, you've probably seen low-calorie foods advertised on television and in magazines as though low-calorie foods were best. It's true that the developed nations of the world have a problem with obesity; in other words, people are eating too many calories. But calories themselves aren't bad for you. Your body needs calories for energy. It's only when you eat more calories than you burn off through activity that you begin to gain weight.

Most foods and drinks contain calories. Some foods, such as celery and lettuce, contain a very few calories. Other foods, like peanuts and sugary foods, contain a lot of calories. The nutrition facts labels on food will tell you how many calories are found in the foods you purchase at the store.

The human body comes in many sizes, and each body burns energy at a different rate; this means that everyone needs a different number of calories to be healthy. The recommended calorie range for most teenagers is 1,600 to 3,000 per day. Boys usually need more than girls, and

Did You Know?

Regular weight gain is the most important sign that a child is developing and growing the way he should. Health-care workers usually weigh children regularly. If a child does not gain weight for two months, he may need more food or different types of food than what he is currently getting.

Did You Know?

Breast-feeding is the best way to make sure a baby's nutritional needs are being met during the first six months of life. Children who are breast-fed receive exactly the right amount of nutrients in the right proportions.

people who are very active will need more calories than those who exercise less.

Protein

Most people need about 1 gram (or a third of an ounce) of protein per kilogram of body mass (or about 0.4 grams of protein per pound of body weight)—so if you weigh 50 kilograms (110 pounds), you'll need to eat about 50 grams of protein each day. As a general rule, between 10 and 15 percent of your total calories should come from protein, which means if you eat 2,000 calories per day, at least 200 should come from protein. When you eat a balanced diet, it's easy to get the protein you need, but for various reasons, not everyone eats a balanced diet. Junk foods like chips, cookies, and other snacks are low in protein, so people who get most of their daily calories from these

Many people in the world's developed nations take for granted that a meal contains protein (meat), carbohydrates (potatoes), and vitamins (green vegetables or tomatoes). In developing nations, however, a meal may be only a carbohydrate such as rice.

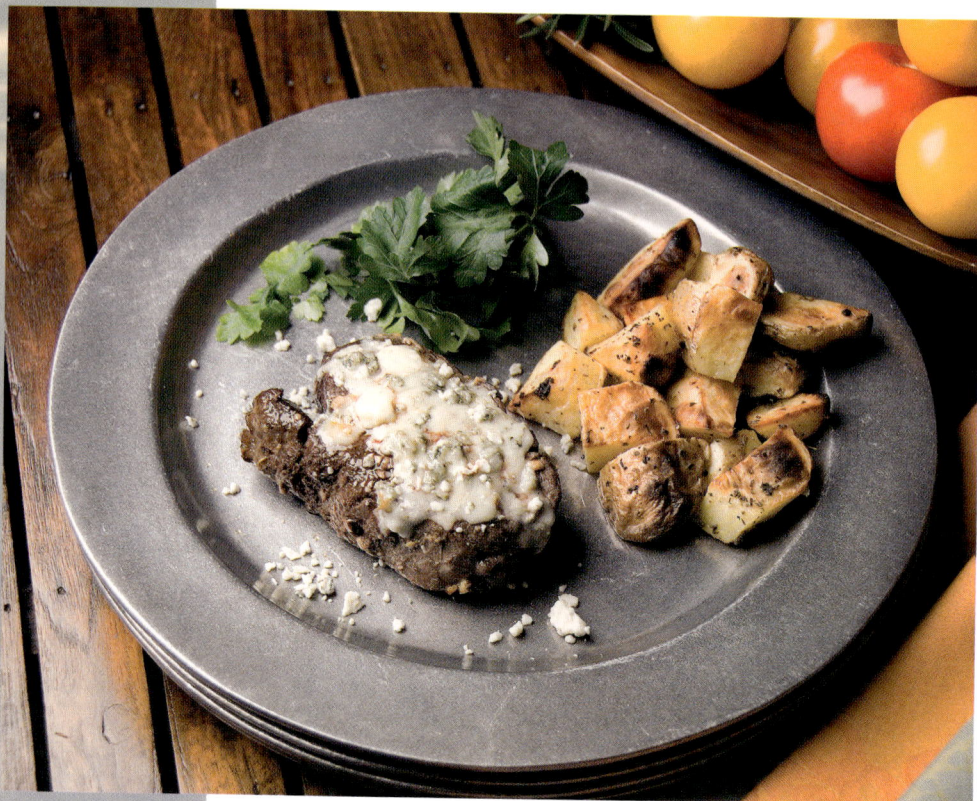

sorts of food may not be eating enough protein. Meanwhile, for many people who live in the developing world, foods that contain protein are expensive and less plentiful than other foods.

Amino acids are the building blocks of protein. The combination of amino acids is what determines the type of protein. There are two types of protein—animal and plant—but there are about 20 different amino acids, divided between essential amino acids and nonessential ones. Essential means the body cannot make these chemicals on its own and must obtain them from a food source. Good nutrition includes all the amino acids, because your body needs them all in order to be healthy.

Depending on the **composition** of amino acids, proteins are either "complete" or "incomplete." Animal protein has all the amino acids your body needs, so beef, chicken, pork, fish, and eggs are all complete proteins. Vegetable proteins—from nuts, seeds, and **legumes**—are usually incomplete, which means they are either missing amino acids or they have too few of them to keep up with what your body needs. Vegetable proteins need to be combined with each other, to make sure all your body's amino acid needs are met.

Carbohydrates

The main fuel your body uses to move around comes from carbohydrates. Carbohydrates can be refined (simple) and unrefined. Refined sugars (like those found in soft drinks, snack foods, and white bread) have already been broken down by food processing; in other words, machinery has removed all the bits of **fiber** from the food. Often, refined sugars have been added to the food, instead of being a natural part of it (as is the case with fruit and vegetables). Your body has to work harder to get the energy from unrefined carbohydrates, and these more **complex** carbohydrates are better for you. Good nutrition requires more complex carbohydrates and as little refined carbohydrates as possible.

Whole-grain breads are better for you than white bread. Whole grains have more fiber and complex carbohydrates.

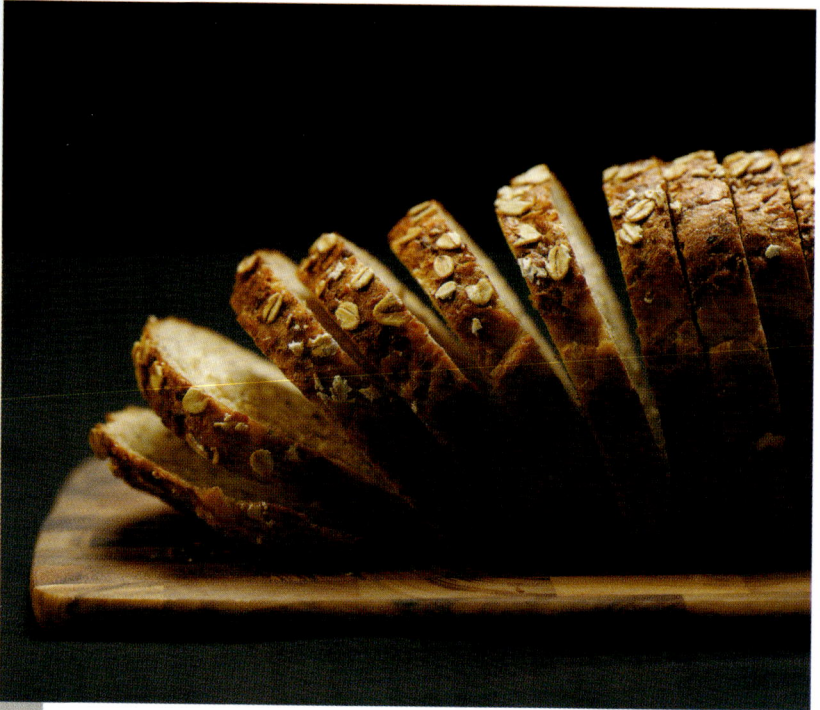

Fats

In many developed countries, fat is talked about as though it were something bad, something we all ought to avoid if at all possible. Although it's true that a high-fat diet is unhealthy and can contribute to a variety of diseases (including heart disease and obesity-related conditions), here's the truth: we need fat in our diets. The right kind of fat in the right amounts is good for you. It provides calories that give the body energy; it helps absorb some vitamins; fat makes up the building blocks of hormones, special chemicals that give directions to your body; and it insulates your body's nervous system tissue. What's more, fat in food helps people feel satisfied, so they end up not eating as many calories.

Fat is a normal part of food. Some foods, including most fruits and vegetables, have almost no fat, while other foods, including oils, nuts, and many meats, have plenty of fat. You need to eat fat every day to be healthy. Teenagers and adults need to get about 30 percent of their daily calories from fat. This means that if you eat about 2,000 calories every day, 600 of those calories should come from fat.

Unsaturated fat is the kind of fat that is best for you. It is found in plant foods and fish. Olive oil, peanut oil, canola oil, albacore tuna, and salmon are all good sources of unsaturated fat.

Saturated fats are found in meat and other animal products, such as dairy products (except those made from skim milk). Saturated fats are also in palm and coconut oils, which are often used in the baked goods you buy at the store. Eating too much saturated fat can increase your risk of heart disease.

Trans fats are found in margarine, especially the sticks, and in many of the snack foods, baked goods, and fried foods you buy at stores and restaurants. Trans fats are also listed on the food label. Like saturated fats, trans fats can raise cholesterol and increase the risk of heart disease.

Vitamins

Your body doesn't need large quantities of vitamins as it does proteins, carbohydrates, and fats, but if you don't get enough of the right vitamins, your nutrition will suffer—and you will not function as well either mentally or physi-

Did You Know?

A calorie is a unit used to measure food's energy. When we're talking about nutrition, the word "calorie" is usually used instead of the more precise scientific term "kilocalorie," which is the amount of energy required to raise the temperature of a liter of water one degree centigrade at sea level. Most people say "calorie" when they're talking about food energy, but it is actually a kilocalorie: 1000 true calories of energy.

Sample Meal with the Right Percentage of Fat

Two slices of bread = 13% fat (30 of 230 calories from fat)
Two tablespoons of peanut butter = 75% fat (140 of 190 calories from fat)
One tablespoon of jelly = 0% fat (0 of 50 calories from fat)
One cup of 1% milk = 18 % (20 of 110 calories from fat)
Apple = 0% (0 of 80 calories from fat)
Total = 29% fat (190 of 660 calories from fat)

Did You Know?

Each gram of carbohydrate or protein provides the body with 4 calories, while each gram of fat provides 9 calories.

Did You Know?

An easy way to figure out how much protein you need is to take your weight in pounds, divide it in half, and subtract 10. The total will be the number of grams of protein you should eat each day. For concentrated proteins such as meat, a 4-ounce serving (about 125 grams) is about the size of a computer mouse or your fist.

cally. Your body does not make vitamins, so you have to get them from food. If you do not have enough of one vitamin, that can also affect your body's ability to absorb other vitamins. Each vitamin has a role to play to keep us healthy.

Vitamins that are fat **soluble** can be stored in your body for a while, some for days, others for months; this means your body can build up a supply to keep on hand for when they are needed. Vitamins A, D, E, and K are fat-soluble. Meanwhile, water-soluble vitamins—vitamins C and B—travel through your bloodstream to your kidneys, where they pass into your urine, and eventually leave your body when you go to the toilet. Your body uses what it needs while the vitamins are traveling through your system. Since you don't have the ability to store them for later, these vitamins need to be replaced often (by eating foods that contain them).

Here are some of the most important vitamins your body needs for good nutrition:

- *The B vitamins* (found in beans, peas, and whole-grain foods) help your body make energy. They support the creation of red blood cells, which carry oxygen around your body.

- *Vitamin C* (found in oranges and other citrus fruit, tomatoes, cabbage, and red and green peppers) helps your body's tissues (for example, skin and muscles) keep healthy. It also helps cuts and wounds to heal and helps you ward off illnesses.

- *Vitamin D* (found in milk, eggs, and salmon) helps you build strong bones and teeth by helping you take in the calcium you need. Regular sunlight helps your body take in vitamin D, but people who live in certain areas of the world may not be exposed to sunshine for long periods of the year. Many developed nations **fortify** milk with vitamin D.

- *Vitamin E* (found in nuts, spinach, and sardines) helps keep body tissues such as your eyes and skin healthy. It also protects your lungs from being damaged by polluted air, and it helps in the making of red blood cells.

- *Vitamin K* (found in liver, pork, and yoghurt) helps your blood clot when you bleed, so that the blood flow does not continue. Some foods with vitamin K include pork, liver and yoghurt.

- *Vitamin A* (found in carrots, pumpkin, yellow squash, apricots, and eggs) is good for your eyes. It helps you be able to see better at night, and it also helps you see colors. A severe lack of vitamin A can even cause blindness. Few people have such an extreme lack of vitamin A; they may not even notice that they aren't

If you eat a variety of vegetables each day, you can be sure you're getting all the vitamins your body needs.

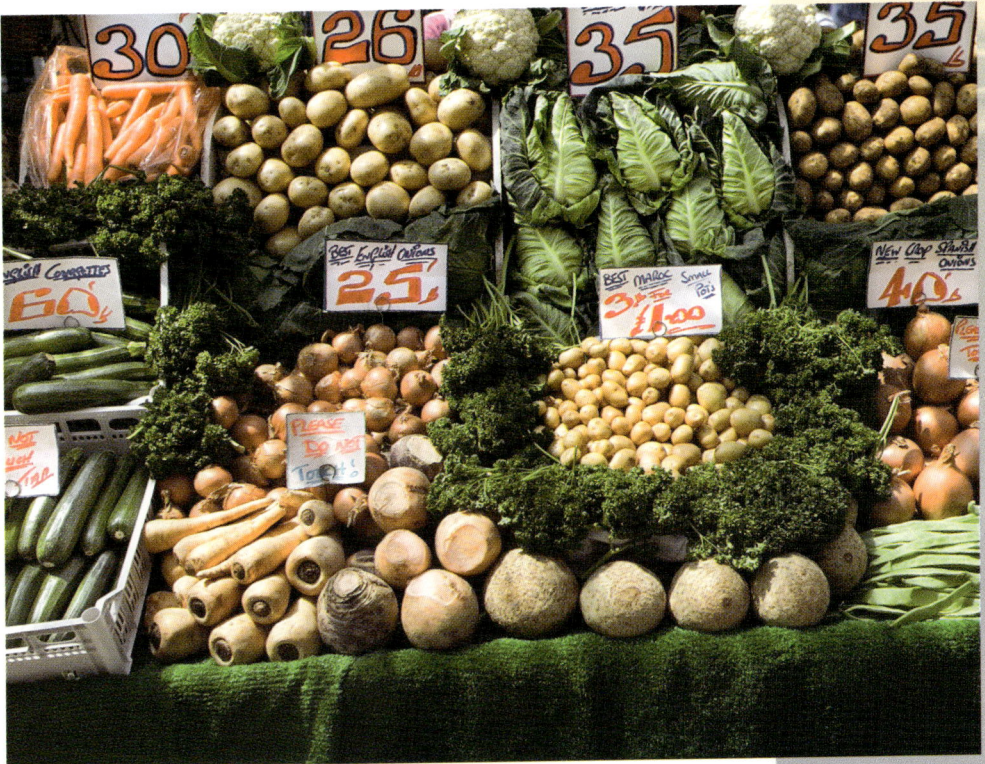

getting enough of this vitamin, but their ability to fight off diseases will be decreased.

Minerals

Minerals are the chemicals found in metals and in the soil. It may seem strange that your body needs something like iron (the same substance that's use to manufacture steel for cars and machinery) or copper (found in coins and cooking pots)—but it does! Your body needs only very tiny bits of minerals like these, but those tiny bits are important for good nutrition. You don't eat coins or metal pots, of course (and too much of many minerals could be dangerous to your health), so how do you get minerals inside your body?

First, plants take in minerals from the soil—and you get those minerals from eating plants. Animals also eat the plants, and the minerals enter their bodies, so you can also get some minerals from eating meat. Minerals can be present in water as well. How much and what minerals you take into our bodies will depend on how much of a mineral is present in the soil in the region where your food, water, or meat comes from. Many developed nations add minerals to their foods, so not getting enough of these substances is seldom a concern, so long as you're eating a

Water

Anything that's alive—from tiny one-celled creatures to human beings to trees—needs water in order to live. Water makes up more than half of a human's body weight and a person can't survive for more than a few days without it. When your body doesn't have enough water, that's called being dehydrated. Low-level dehydration can affect your body and mind's performance, while a bad case of dehydration can make you sick. When your urine is very dark yellow, it's means your body is holding on to water, so it's probably time to drink more. You need extra water when you exercise and when it's hot out. People who live in developed nations may take water for granted (turn on the faucet and out it comes), but people who live in other regions of the world may have to walk long distances and carry water back to their home.

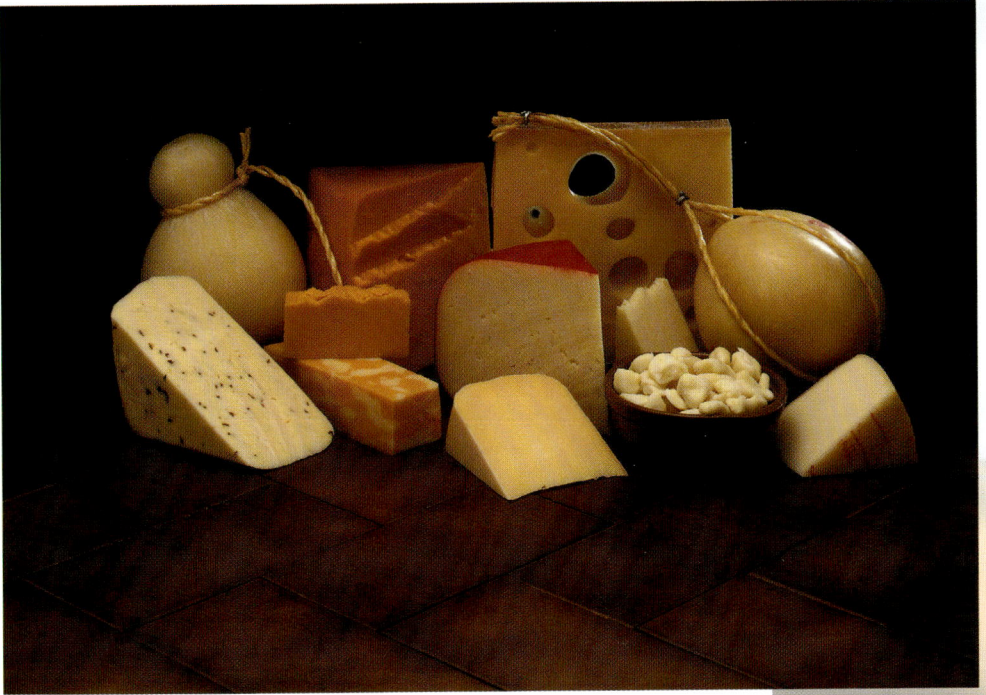

balanced diet—but if you live in a **developing** nation, you may be dependent on the food that grows on the land where you live, which may or may not have all the minerals you need for good nutrition.

Here are some of the minerals most important to good nutrition:

- *Calcium* (found in dairy products, tofu, and cabbage) is needed to help build your bones and teeth.

- *Sodium* (the mineral found in salt) helps regulate the fluid balance in your body; it also helps your muscles expand (stretch) and contract (get smaller), which is what allows your body to move. Salt is present in all your body's fluids, including tears and sweat. You may have heard that a low-salt diet is often considered to be healthy, and too much salt can cause high-blood pressure—but not enough salt can also be dangerous to your health.

All kinds of cheese are good sources of protein and calcium. Many of them also have high levels of saturated fat, though, so you need to be careful of how much you eat.

• *Iron* (found in dark, leafy vegetables and peanuts) helps your brain develop normally.

• *Iodine* is also important for normal brain development. A lack of iodine can cause goiters (where a part of the body called the thyroid gland becomes larger), hearing and speaking difficulty, and poor growth. The world's developed nations add iodine to their salt to make sure that people get enough of this mineral, and nearly two-thirds of the developing nations also add iodine to salt.

Food and Finances

Everyone on Earth needs good nutrition—but not all people get the foods they need to be healthy. Sometimes poor nutrition is caused by bad eating habits, getting too many calories from high-fat, sugary foods that contribute to obesity and don't contain enough of the nutrients our bodies need. In many parts of the world, though, both in developed and developing nations, poor nutrition is linked to poverty. Families that don't have enough money may not be able to afford a healthy variety of foods. In some parts of the world, there simply may not be enough food resources to meet the needs of the communities who live there. Poverty looks different in different parts of the world—but it always has an enormous impact on nutrition.

The Food Pyramid

The United States' Food Guide Pyramid is a picture people use to help them understand how to eat healthy. The colored stripes represent the main food groups.

orange = grains
green = vegetables
red = fruits

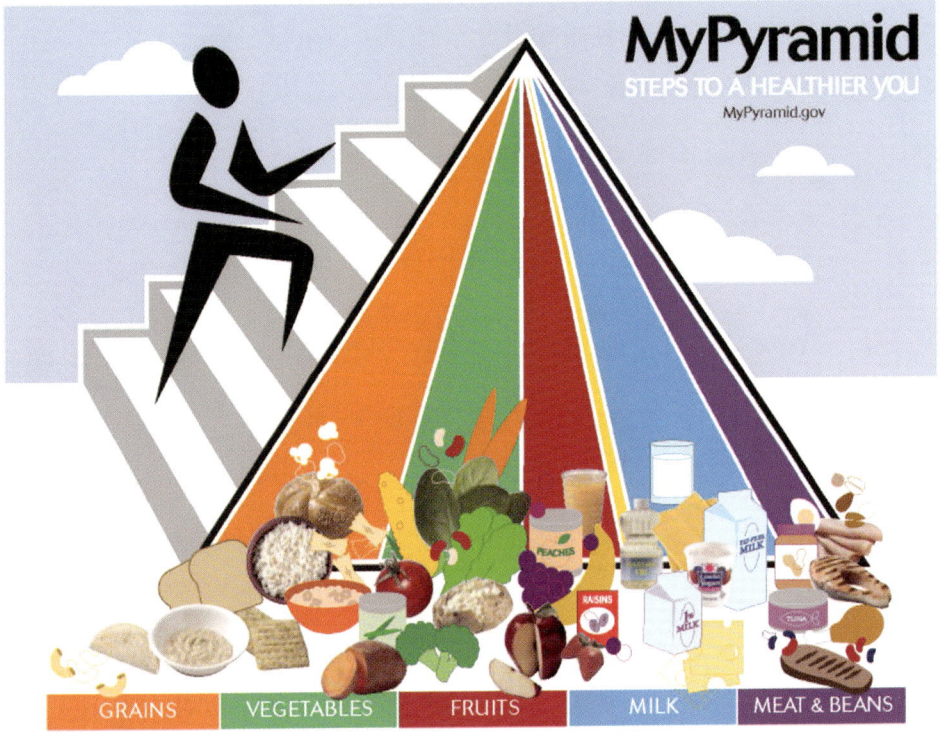

MyPyramid
STEPS TO A HEALTHIER YOU
MyPyramid.gov

GRAINS   VEGETABLES   FRUITS   MILK   MEAT & BEANS

The U.S. Food Pyramid.

yellow = fats and oils
blue = milk and dairy products
purple = meat, beans, fish, and nuts

Here are the important things you should learn from the pyramid:

- **Eat a variety of foods.** A balanced diet is one that includes all the food groups, so eat foods from every color, every day.

- **Eat less of some foods, and more of others.** Notice that the stripes for meat and protein (purple) and oils (yellow) are skinnier than the others. That's because you need less of those foods than you do of fruits, vegetables, grains, and dairy foods. You can also see that the stripes start out wider at the bottom of the pyramid and get thinner as they reach

Did You Know?

Athletes and other people who exercise a lot have different nutritional needs than those who don't. They need both more protein and more carbohydrates.

Nutrition and Health Around the World

• About 30% of children in many developed countries, including Canada, Australia, New Zealand, and the United States, are either overweight or obese as result of poor nutrition habits.

• Over 70% of preschool children in India are estimated to be iron-deficient. (In other words, they don't get enough iron to be healthy.)

• In Canada, fewer than 5% of pregnant women know that vitamin supplements would contribute to the health of their unborn children.

• About 70% of children under 6 in Kenya suffer from vitamin A deficiency.

• As many as 18 million low-birth-weight babies are born every year due to malnutrition; that's 14% of all live births. These children are likely to suffer from infections, weakened immunity, learning disabilities, and impaired physical and mental development.

(Source: UNICEF International Web site)

Did You Know?

Most Americans get about 50 percent of their carbohydrates from simple, refined sugars. Over the course of a year, the average American drinks 54 gallons of soda, which contains the highest amounts of added sugars of any food.

the top. That's meant to show you that not all foods are created equal, even within a healthy food group like fruit. For instance, an apple tart would probably be in that thin part of the fruit stripe because it has added sugar and fat. A whole apple would be down in the wide part because you can eat more of those within a healthy diet.

Global Images for Good Nutrition

Countries around the world use many different methods to get this information to their citizens. For instance, a rainbow symbolizes Canadian guidelines. Among its recommendations are to eat five to twelve servings of grains and up to ten daily servings of fruits and vegetables. They also advise moderation in the use of caffeine. Costa Rica's nutritional guidelines are presented on a plate, and they advise that foods be consumed in the most natural form possible. Australia and Great Britain also use plates as

Vegetarians must eat "complementary" vegetable proteins to make a single complete protein source. For example, they need to eat beans with rice—or a rice cake with peanut butter or hummus (made from seeds). Soy is a good low-fat source of protein for vegetarians. Most protein bars and protein powders use soy protein, casein, or whey as their base, which are all are complete proteins. Whey, however, is a milk product, so if you are a vegan, you may want to avoid products that contain whey.

Health Canada **Santé Canada**

CANADA'S Food Guide

TO HEALTHY EATING
FOR PEOPLE FOUR YEARS AND OVER

Enjoy a variety of foods from each group every day.

Choose lower-fat foods more often.

Grain Products
Choose whole grain and enriched products more often.

Vegetables and Fruit
Choose dark green and orange vegetables and orange fruit more often.

Milk Products
Choose lower-fat milk products more often.

Meat and Alternatives
Choose leaner meats, poultry and fish, as well as dried peas, beans and lentils more often.

Canada

Health Canada's Food Rainbow.

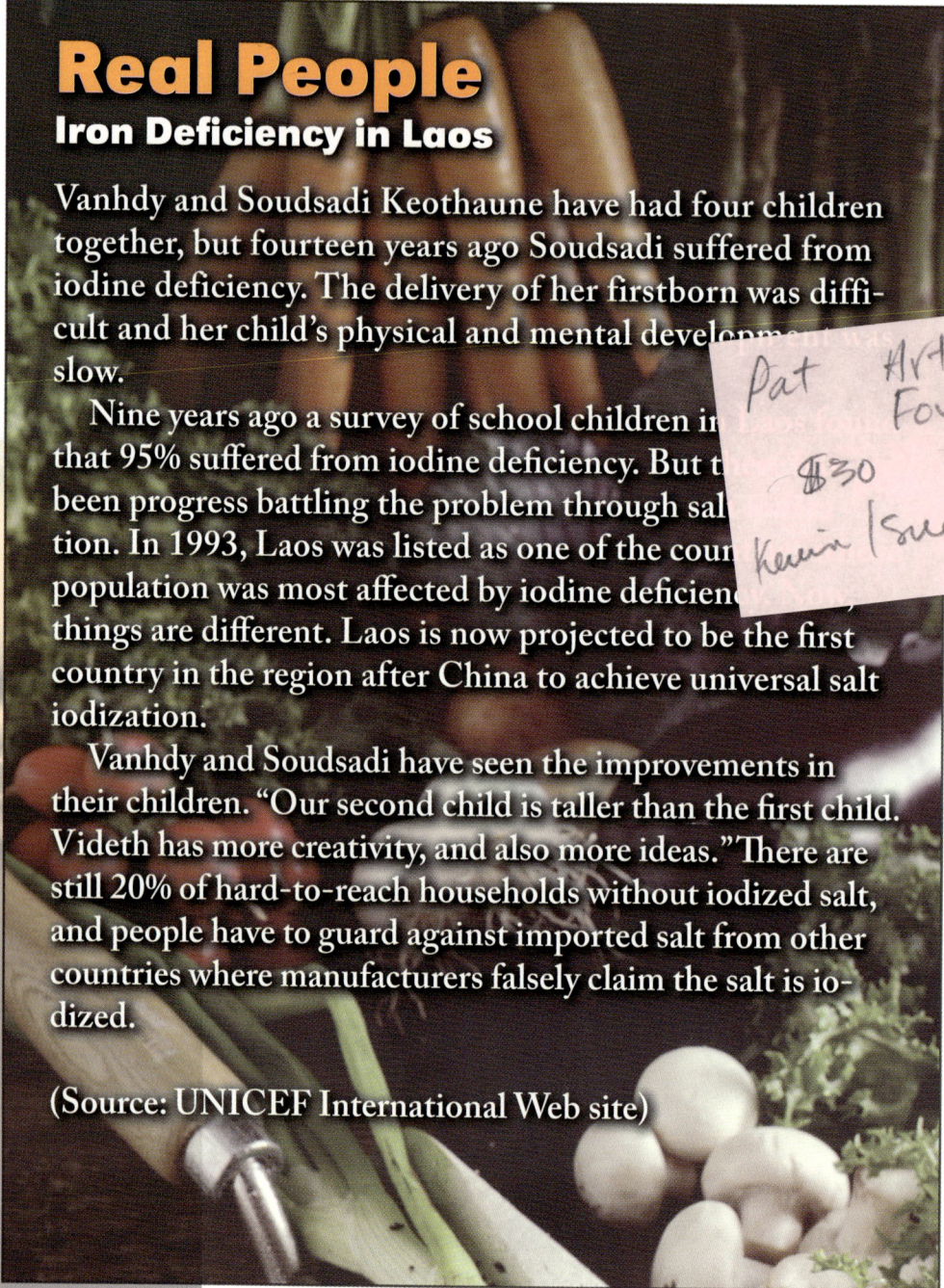

Real People
Iron Deficiency in Laos

Vanhdy and Soudsadi Keothaune have had four children together, but fourteen years ago Soudsadi suffered from iodine deficiency. The delivery of her firstborn was difficult and her child's physical and mental development was slow.

Nine years ago a survey of school children in Laos found that 95% suffered from iodine deficiency. But there has been progress battling the problem through salt iodization. In 1993, Laos was listed as one of the countries whose population was most affected by iodine deficiency. Today, things are different. Laos is now projected to be the first country in the region after China to achieve universal salt iodization.

Vanhdy and Soudsadi have seen the improvements in their children. "Our second child is taller than the first child. Videth has more creativity, and also more ideas." There are still 20% of hard-to-reach households without iodized salt, and people have to guard against imported salt from other countries where manufacturers falsely claim the salt is iodized.

(Source: UNICEF International Web site)

Japan's Spinning Food Top.

Spinning speed of the top shows the level of physical activity.

Physical Activity

The top axis shows water or teas. Be careful to have enough water during meal.

Grain dishes
(Rice, Bread, Noodles, and Pasta)

Vegetable dishes

The top itself shows a well-balanced diet.

Fish and Meat dishes
(Meat, Fish, Egg and Soy-bean dishes)

Enjoy Snacks, Confection and Beverages moderately!

The top falls due to unbalanced diet or lack of physical activity.

Milk
(Milk and Milk products)

It is important to enjoy snacks, confection and beverages moderately.

Fruits

Spin the top of balanced diet!

their food guide visual aide. A spinning top is the nutritional symbol of Japan's guidelines. According to Japanese guidelines, happy eating means a happy family life, and they encourage family meal preparation and eating. Variety is also important in the Japanese diet, and the guidelines recommend consuming thirty different foods every day.

Did You Know?

Getting enough iron is especially important for children between the ages of six months and two years. In developed countries, many infant foods such as cereals have added iron, and 49 of the world's countries fortify their flour with iron.

STRAIGHT FROM THE SOURCE

(by Kent Page, UNICEF)

Community Gardens Provide Food, Income for Families

AGADEZ, Niger, 14 September 2005—Niger is struggling to cope with a nutrition crisis. But in the village of Alikinkin, community gardens are an oasis of beauty and a source of food, helping children avoid the worst effects of the crisis.

In Alikinkin's gardens, donkeys, goats and birds flourish among the grasses, bushes, palm and date trees. Neatly planted rows of crops are irrigated with fresh water pumped from wells—a stark contrast to the situation in other parts of the country.

UNICEF's office in Agadez, a town near Alikinkin, is supporting 50 community garden projects by helping construct water wells, providing gardening seeds, fertilizer, insecticide, fencing and tools.

The goal is to ensure that village children have access to nutritious foods. The gardens produce tomatoes, onions, carrots, peas, beans, cabbage, potatoes and wheat.

What Do You Think?

• How are gardens and nutrition connected?

• Do you think your nutrition concerns are similar to those of the people who live in Alikinkin in Niger? Why or why not?

• Do you think it would be better if developed nations merely shipped their excess food to Niger (instead of helping to build gardens) to ensure good nutrition for communities like Alikinkin? Why or why not?

Find Out More

Food Guidelines by Country
http://www.fao.org/ag/agn/nutrition/education_
guidelines_country_en.stm

MyPyramid
www.mypyramid.gov

U.S. Department of Agriculture, Center for Nutrition Policy and Promotion
www.cnpp.usda.gov

Here's what you need to know

- **Poverty means not having the basic things necessary for life.**
- **The World Bank defines poverty as earning $2US or less a day, and extreme poverty as less than $1 a day.**
- **Poverty limits people's choices.**
- **People living in poverty are at greater risk for other problems.**
- **Poverty is a global problem.**
- **Five main factors contribute to poverty:**
  - **educational opportunities**
  - **business opportunities**
  - **environmental conditions**
  - **government**
  - **health care**

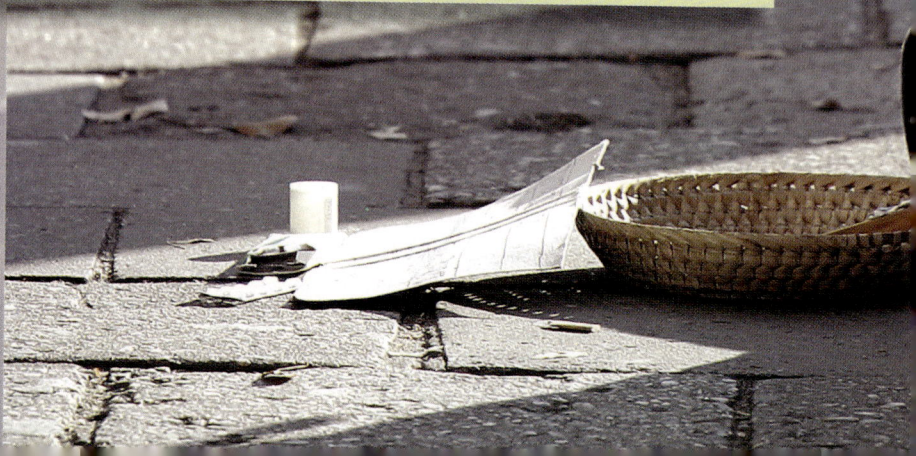

Words to Understand

Deprivation is a state of loss, of doing without.

Sanitation facilities are the services that promote good health and hygiene by removing garbage, sewage, and other waste products from the community in a safe way.

Empowerment is the gift of power, which includes the ability to make choices, to be all that a person can be.

Vulnerability is a state of being open to physical or emotional pain or damage.

Something that is **corrupt** lacks a sense of right and wrong; it is rotten in a moral sense.

Transitioning means moving from one condition to another.

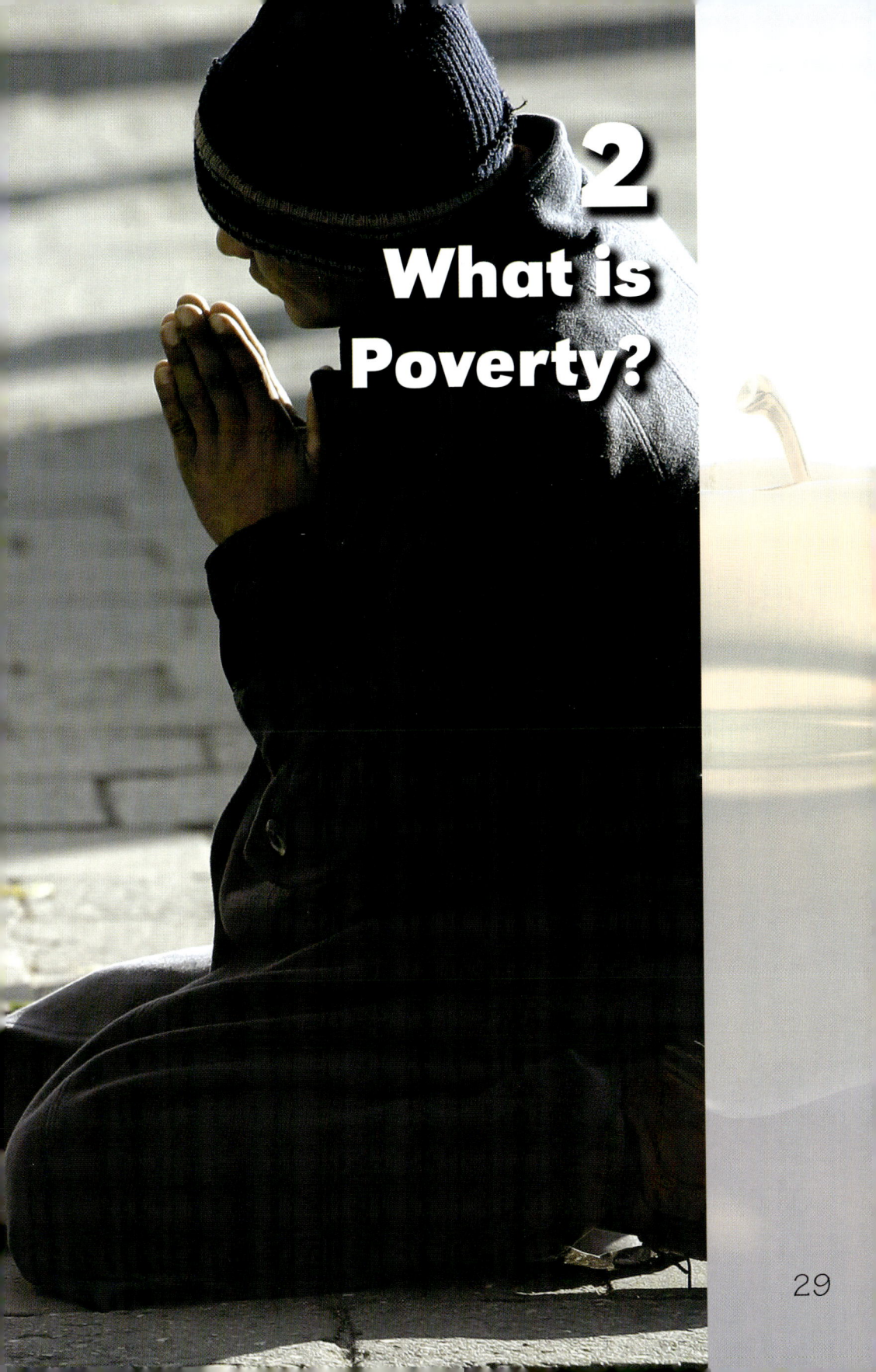

2
What is Poverty?

People who are poor don't have much money, right? But it's not as simple as that. People living in poverty lack many of the basic things a lot of us take for granted. The United Nations defines poverty as "a condition characterised by severe **deprivation** of basic human needs, including food, safe drinking water, **sanitation facilities**, health, shelter, education, and information." When people don't have enough to eat, when their children can't go to school,

Poverty is when you don't have enough of the basic things you need: food, clothing, housing, education. If you gave this child a check for a million dollars, would he be rich—or would he still be poor? What do you think?

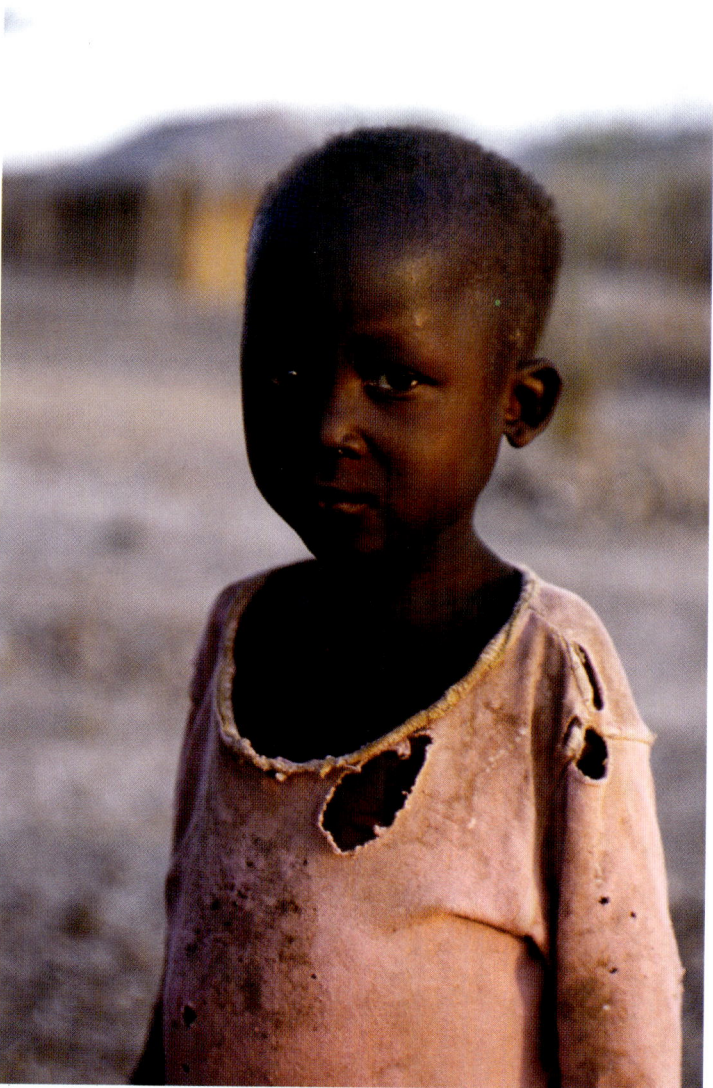

or when they don't have health care, then they can be considered to be living in poverty, regardless of their income. After all, what good is a hundred-dollar bill if you don't have anything you can buy with it?

How Governments Define Poverty

It's useful for governments to be able to say exactly what poverty is. That way they can think about what they need to and how much money they'll need to spend to fix the problem. These definitions help governments decide who gets government help and who doesn't.

Sometimes governments say that poverty includes everyone who is in the 10 percent of people with the lowest incomes. This may work in a country like the United States or the United Kingdom, where the overall incomes are relatively high—but it doesn't work in a country like the Sudan, where even the highest incomes are very low by U.S. or UK standards. And it doesn't work in a country like Peru, where a very small segment of the nation have very, very high incomes, while the rest of the country has very small incomes.

Another way governments may define poverty is by figuring out exactly how much money people need to buy life's most basic requirements: food, shelter, water. The World Bank has come up with a global definition of poverty that says that around the world, people need at least $2US per day in order to buy life's basic needs. This means that anyone who makes less than $750 in a year would be considered to be living in poverty. People who make $1 a day (or $365 a year) or less are considered to be living in extreme poverty.

This number doesn't make sense for developed countries, though, where the cost of living is much higher. No one in the United States, for example, would try to live on $750 a year! In the United States, the poverty line for 2005 was set at $26.19 a day (or about $9550 a year).

Did You Know?

Half the world— that's about 3 billion people— live on less than $3US.

Did You Know?

Using the World Bank's definition of poverty, 2.7 billion people lived in poverty in 2005, and 1.1 billion people lived in extreme poverty. Most of these people live in Africa or South Asia.

Other Definitions of Poverty

Not everyone agrees that poverty can be defined using numbers and statistics. According to Kathleen McHugh from Save the Children, "Poverty should be defined by a person's inability [to bring about] change in their lives." Experts call this concept empowerment. It refers to people's ability to make choices for themselves.

For instance, imagine you have a million dollars—but you're on a deserted island, with no stores, no people, no anything. What choices do you have? Or imagine that you have a million dollars in the bank—but you're 85 years old, you're sick and weak, you can't get to the store, you don't know how to use the Internet, and you have no one to take care of you. What choices do you have? Now imagine that you have a million dollars—but you live in a country where people who look like you aren't allowed to go into certain stores, attend certain schools, or even talk to certain people. What choices do you have? Poverty is more complicated than how much money you have in the bank!

That's why sometimes governments and experts may define poverty by comparing the richest people in a nation to the poorest people. In the European Union (EU), for example, the poverty line is set at 60 percent of the average income. In the UK, where the average income is about $34,000US, the poverty line would be about $20,000US. Obviously, the people living below this line are nowhere near as poor as people living in many African countries, for example—but compared to other people in their society, the people below this line have fewer choices available to them. Their low income puts walls around their lives, limiting where they can live, where they can go, the jobs they can get, the kind of health care they have, and how they interact with others in their society.

Vulnerability

When experts talk about vulnerability in connection to poverty, they mean that people who are poor are at greater risk for other problems as well. People who have less money have fewer resources to fall back on should a disaster occur (whether that disaster is caused by nature, their health, or the government). For instance, if you live in a poor family in Guatemala, your family may depend on the money that comes from the crops your father grows on a small farm. Now imagine that your father gets sick. Your family has no safety net. You become even poorer than you were before. You and your older brothers and sisters stay home from school so you can work on the farm. This means that when you grow up, you will not be able to get a good-paying job, and you will probably be as poor as your parents are. Suppose your mother gets sick. That means there is no one to take care of your little brothers, so you stay home to watch them—but now there are fewer hands to work the farm, and it produces even less food. Your parents need medicine, but there is not enough money even to feed the family, let alone buy medicine. And finally, imagine that a hurricane sweeps through your

Disasters such as fires and floods can plunge people into poverty, leaving them without homes, clothing, or other belongings, forcing them to take refuge in temporary shelters like this.

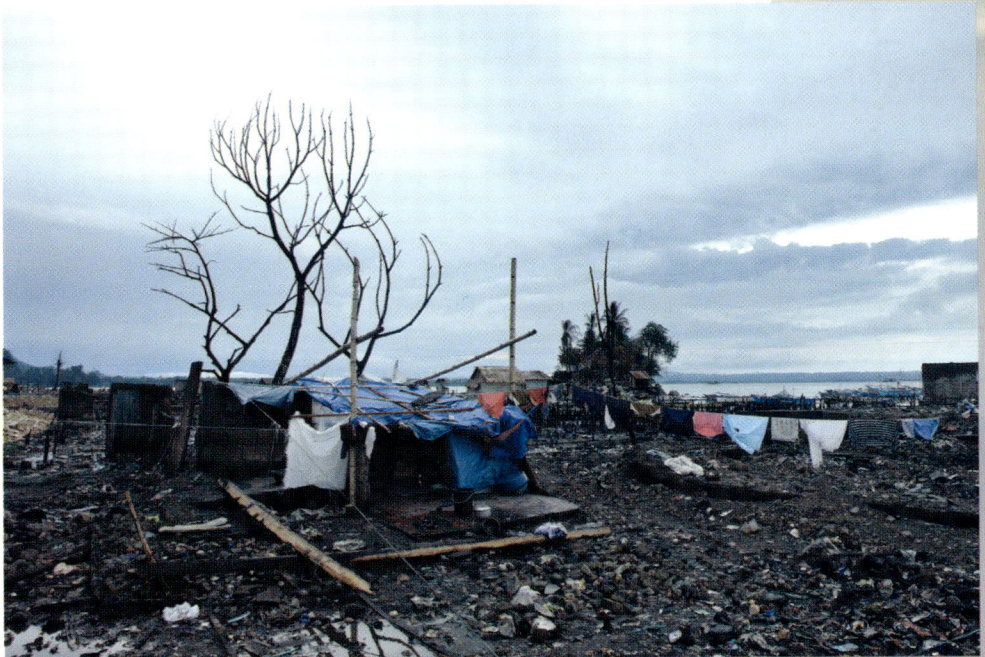

community, destroying your house and all the crops. Now what do you do?

Poverty puts people at risk for many dangers.

A Global Problem

Poverty circles the globe. Even the richest nations have their share of people who do not have the same opportunities for nutrition, education, and good health. But poverty is a far more desperate problem in the world's developing nations. The following regions are particularly at risk:

• *Sub-Sahara Africa.* This term refers to the portion of Africa that lies south of the Sahara desert—and it is one of the poorest regions on our planet. Almost 50 percent of the population there lives on under $1US a day; this is the highest rate of extreme poverty in the world. Thirty-two of the world's 48 poorest countries are located in this region. Their people's lives are made worse by ongoing wars and political conflicts, unstable and corrupt governments, and terrible diseases, including malaria and HIV/AIDS. In the last 25 years, the number of people living in poverty in this region has doubled.

• *Southeast Asia.* After sub-Sahara Africa, Southeast Asia is probably the poorest region, with about half of the world's poor living there. In a population of 1.3 billion, 85 percent (more than a billion people) live on less than $2 a day.

• *Eastern Asia and Pacific.* This region is home to nearly 2 billion people, making it one of the most populated regions on earth. About 50 percent of the population lives on less than $2US a day. China, however, makes up a huge part of this region, and in the past few years, this nation has made huge economic and social advances; this means that the number of people living in poverty in the region has

dropped greatly. The situation in China continues to improve, even as the overall population continues to grow.

- *North Africa and the Middle East.* About 23 percent of the population in North Africa and the Middle East live on less than $2 a day, but only 2.2 percent (6 million people) live on under $1 a day. However, many of countries in the region depend almost

This woman and her children live in Myanmar in Southeast Asia, one of the world's poorest regions.

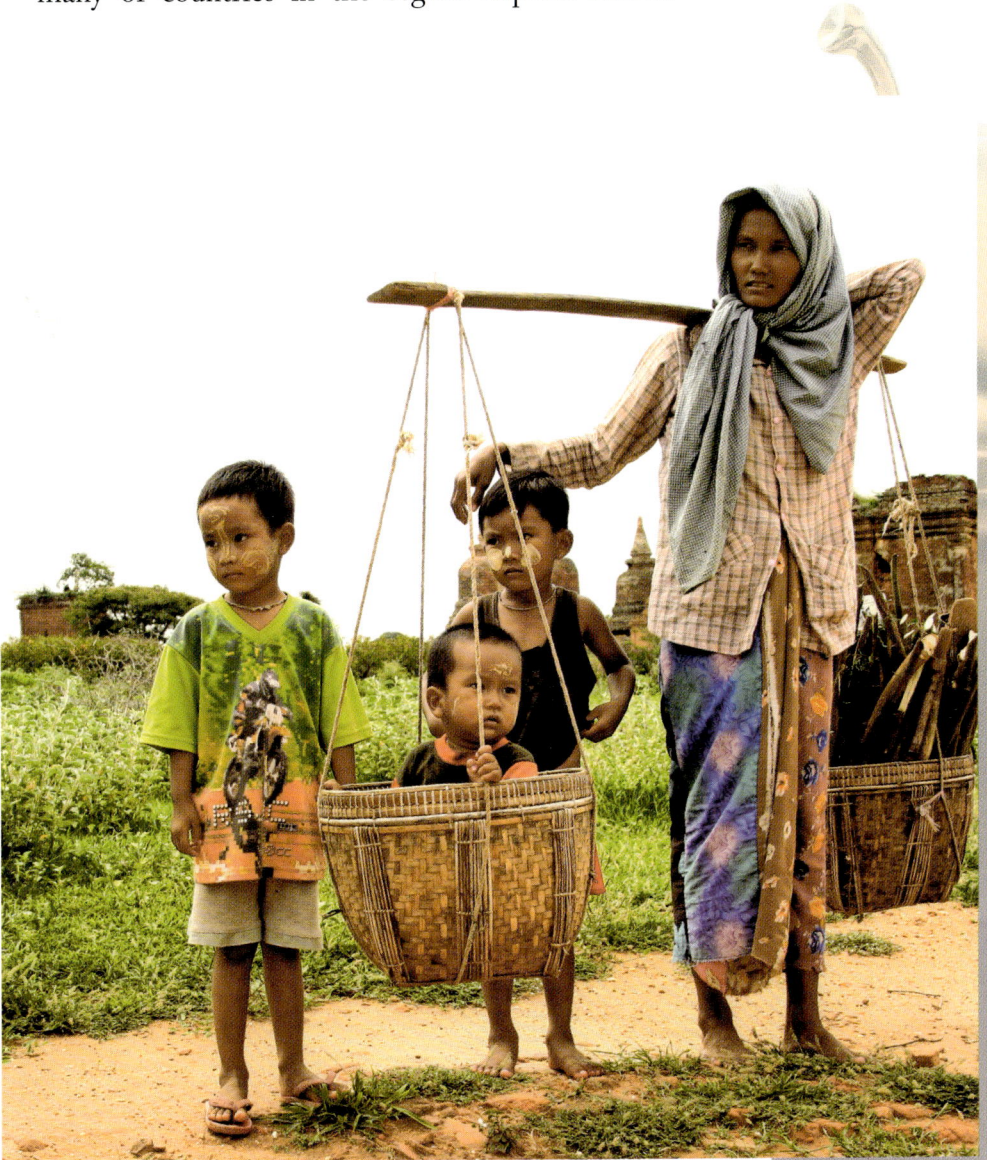

Medical care in the Sudan, like in much of Africa and other developing regions of the world, is often not easily available. People may have to walk long distances to see a doctor and medicines are very expensive.

completely on one product—oil—for their wealth. What will happen to these countries as the world shifts to other energy sources?

• *Latin America.* Of the approximately 534 million people living in Latin America, 132 million live on less than $2US a day, and 57 million live on less than $1US a day. The situation is improving, but income levels in this region are still very unequal. According to the World Bank, "the richest one-tenth of the population of Latin America and the Caribbean earn 48 percent of total income, while the poorest

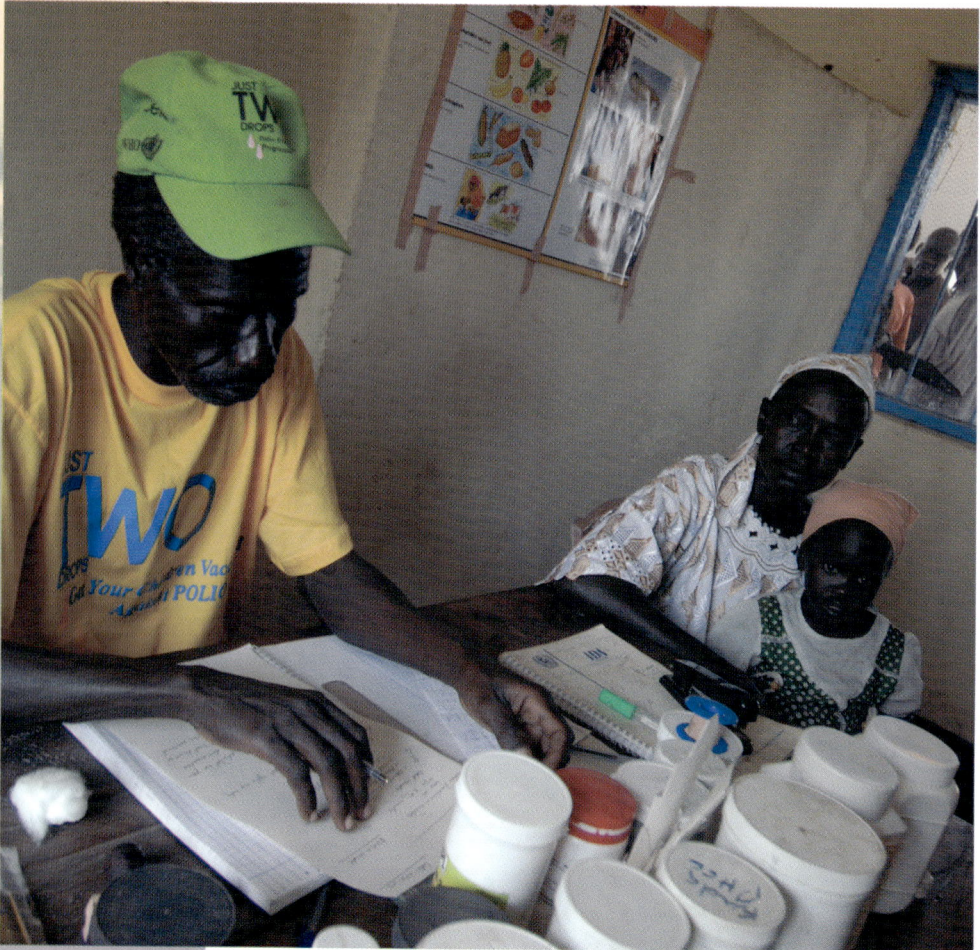

tenth earn only 1.6 percent." That means if you were cutting up a pie, half of it would be divided between 53 million rich people, while only a tiny sliver of the pie would be passed out to 53 million poor people.

• *Eastern Europe and Central Asia.* Much of this region was once a part of the old Soviet Republic; when the Soviet government fell in 1991, the new countries that were born faced many problems. With a population of around 471 million people, 20.3 percent (97 million people), live on less than $2 a day, and 24 million live on less than $1 a day. The situation is rapidly improving in these countries, however, as many are being accepted into the European Union, and the region's economy is growing steadily. Between 1999 and 2003, 40 million people in this region escaped poverty. The nations of Eastern Europe and Central Asia are sometimes regarded as **transitioning** countries, meaning that they are moving from poverty to better circumstances.

Meanwhile, in the developed nations of the world, a segment of the population also lives in poverty. The situation may not be as desperate as it is in other regions, but these people nevertheless face challenges and hardships. According to the U.S. Department of Agriculture, for example, 11 percent of the households in the United States in 2002 faced what experts call "food insecurity"; in other words, they didn't have enough food to offer all household members an active, healthy life. Using educational opportunities as another standard for poverty, the UN's research shows that in two of the world's most stable and prosperous nations—the United States and the United

Ask the Doctor

Q: How come the poor kids in school have runny noses so often? Why do they smell funny sometimes?

Being poor usually means that children in the family don't eat as well and they probably don't go to the doctor as often. This may make them more apt to get sick with colds and other illnesses. These families also don't have as much money for clothes, so they have fewer clothes, and they probably don't have a washing machine. This may mean they wear their clothing more times before washing it, which can cause odor. Sometimes, low-income housing has inadequate plumbing, which may make it more difficult to take showers and baths. Remember that being poor does not make a person less intelligent, less kind, or less valuable!

Kingdom—about 20 percent of the population cannot read or write; in Italy, 47 percent of the population lack these skills. And if we look at health-care opportunities, we find that in two developed countries—Denmark and the United States—health care is so limited that about 11 percent of the population won't live to be 60 years old.

What Causes Poverty?

You can't point to any one single thing as the reason for poverty around the world. Instead, the reasons vary from

All human beings, including this little girl in India, have the right to be healthy and happy— but poverty may rob her of her most basic rights.

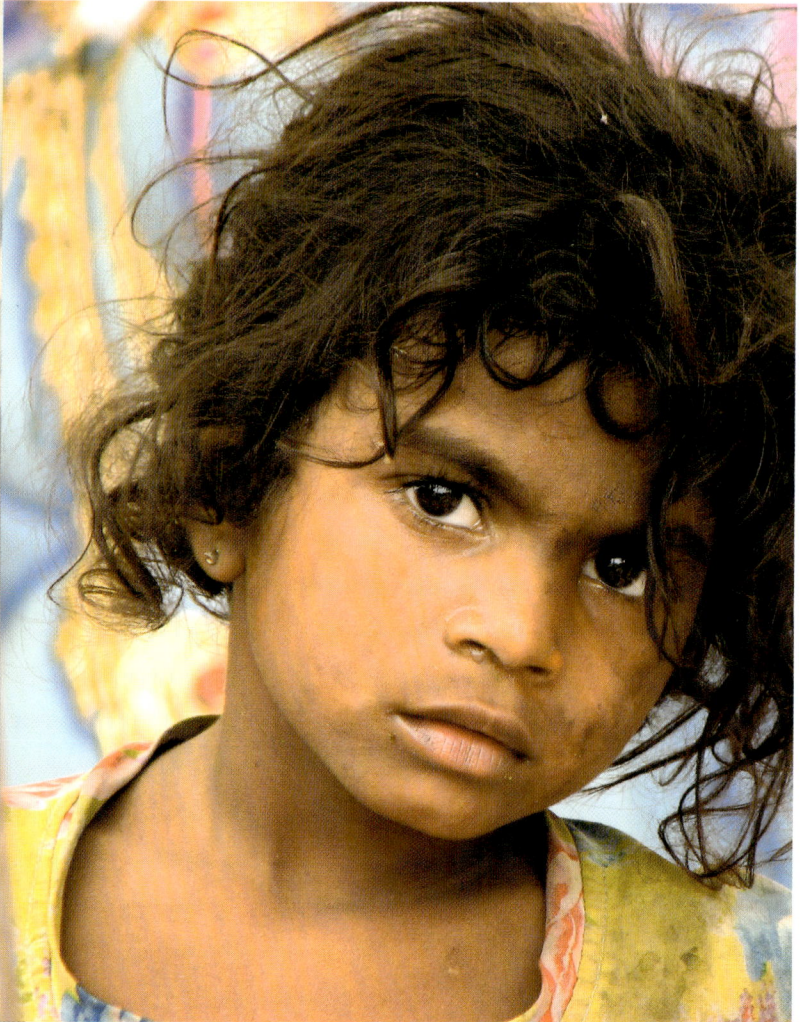

country to country, and from family to family. However, five main factors contribute to poverty all over the globe:

- *Education.* Lack of educational opportunities for children living in poverty means that when they grow up, they will also have fewer professional opportunities. It means they will be less likely to lift themselves out of their family's poverty.

- *Limited business opportunities.* People living in poverty don't have the same opportunities others in the society have for jobs or starting a business—for instance, they do not have access to a loan from a bank or other funding, or there may be fewer jobs available—and without these opportunities, they have no means to change their circumstances.

- *Environmental factors.* Natural disasters, damaged farmland, drought, and lack of natural resources all contribute to a region's poverty level.

- *Government.* Government structures can either help poor people or get in their way. People living in poverty have far fewer opportunities when they live in developing countries where the government doesn't work very well because it is corrupt, weak, or just not very well planned.

- *Health care.* Poor health means wage earners can work less—which in turn means they earn less money, driving their families deeper into poverty. High medical costs can also contribute to poverty. If poor health takes the life of a wage earner, the family is even more at risk for poverty-related dangers.

A Complicated Problem

Sometimes, poverty seems like a fact of life; it's sad, but really, what can we do about it? It's just the way things

Real People

Food Crisis in Niger:

Nana's Battle to Stay Alive

When Nana no longer had the strength to sit up on her own, her parents realized she needed medical care. She was suffering from severe malnutrition. Since there is no health facility in their village her parents had to travel to a therapeutic feeding centre in Maradi the capital of Niger. They knew about the centre because of other children in the village who had been there. They walked by night until they could get to a village where they could get public transport to the capital. Nana started off having therapeutic milk and then moved onto phase two of treatment which included a vitamin rich peanut paste named "Plumpy Nut." Children stay longer in phase two, which consists of four stages called Lions, Tigers, Rhinos and Elephants. After four weeks of help Nana is now an Elephant. In the afternoons the staff of the UNICEF supported centre train mothers and other caregivers in nutrition, health care and sanitation practices.

(Source: UNICEF International Website, Marlene Barger, June 2005)

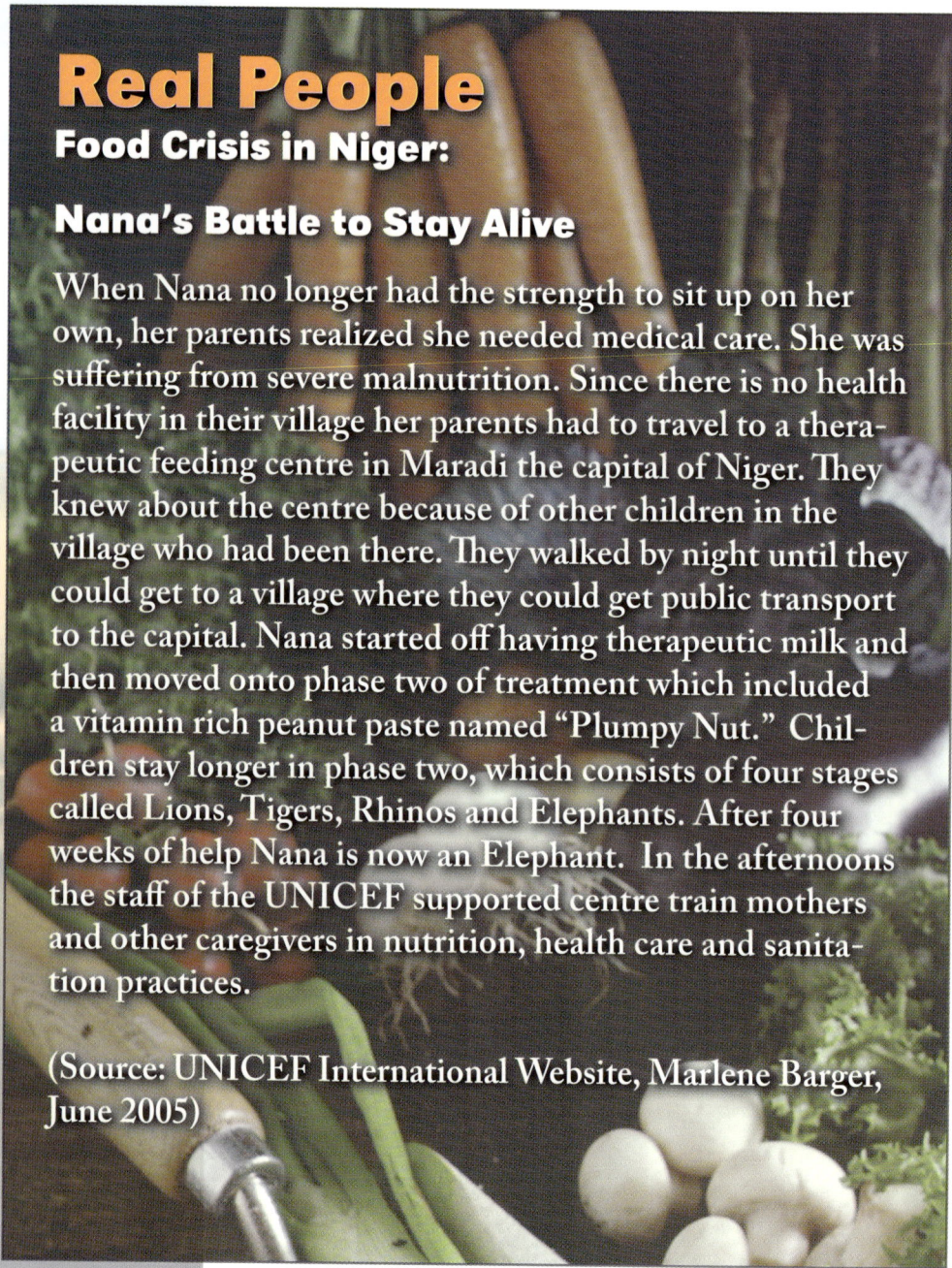

are. In 1948, however, the United Nations' members agreed that all people have the right to education, work, health, and well-being. Poverty keeps people from these most basic rights. In other words, poverty denies human rights.

But it's a big problem. It affects the entire Earth—which means this problem will need all the world's countries to work together to solve it. And because it's such a complicated problem, it needs to be broken down, so that people can work on fixing some of the issues that contribute to poverty around the world. These issues include nutrition, clean water, education, and health care.

In today's world, nutrition is one of the greatest health issues interwoven throughout poverty. Nutrition impacts on many other issues; if you don't have the food you need to function normally, it will be hard for you to go to school and learn, or to hold a job and earn money; if you don't have good nutrition, you will be more vulnerable to diseases; and both of these things will contribute to making you still poorer. Poor nutrition makes poverty worse. And it's a problem that circles the globe.

STRAIGHT FROM THE SOURCE

(From the "State of the World's Children," 2008 UNICEF document.)

The Value of Children

What is a life worth? Most of us would sacrifice a great deal to save a single child. Yet somehow on a global scale, our priorities have become blurred. Every day, on average more than 26,000 children under the age of five die around the world, mostly from preventable causes. Nearly all of them live in the developing world or, more precisely, in 60 developing countries. More than one third of these children die during the first month of life, usually at home and without access to essential health services and basic commodities that might save their lives. . . .

Why child survival matters

Investing in the health of young children makes sense for a number of reasons beyond the pain and suffering caused by even one child's death. Depriving infants and young children of basic health care and denying them the nutrients needed for growth and development sets them up to fail in life. But when children are well nourished and cared for and provided with a safe and stimulating environment, they are more likely to survive, to have less disease and fewer illnesses, and to fully develop thinking, language, emotional and social skills. When they enter school, they are more likely to succeed. And later in life, they have a greater chance of becoming creative and productive members of society.

. . . Improvements in child health and survival can also foster more balanced population dynamics. When parents are convinced that their children will survive, they are more likely to have fewer children and provide better care to those they do have—and countries can invest more in each child.

What Do You Think?

- Why is it easier to ignore the thousands of a children dying each day than it would be a single child in trouble in our front yard? What are some of the reasons for our blindness?

- How does the UNICEF document indicate that the future of the world will be improved if we take care of today's children?

- In a world where people sometimes worry about over population, how does this document indicate that keeping children alive might actually decrease the birth rate?

Find Out More

To find out more about poverty, check out these Web sites:

Causes of Poverty
www.globalissues.org/TradeRelated/Poverty.asp

U.S. Census Bureau, Poverty in the United States
www.census.gov/hhes/www/poverty/poverty.html

World Poverty
www.poverty.com

Words to Understand

A **sub-continent** is a small part of a continent. India is often referred to as a subcontinent because of its size.

Sub-Saharan Africa is the part of Africa that lies south of the Sahara Desert.

Something that is **impaired** has had its strength, usefulness, or health diminished.

Distribution is the process of moving a product from its source to the people who will buy it and use it.

Something that is **inefficient** doesn't produce the desired results, is wasteful, or lacks the ability to perform effectively.

A **famine** is a drastic, wide-reaching food shortage.

A **drought** is a prolonged period of dryness.

Crop yield is the amount of grain or other crop harvested from each planting.

Democracy is government by the people or their elected representatives.

Human rights are the basic freedoms to which all people are entitled.

Social has to do with interactions between people and groups of people.

Political has to do with the structure of government.

To **consolidate** means to unite into one.

Civil refers to anything that applies to ordinary citizens.

Something that is **uncensored** has not been screened and had information removed or hidden by the government (or anyone else).

The **press** refers to newspapers and other news media.

Here's what you need to know

- **Millions of people are starving in the world's developing nations.**
- **Malnutrition is a less urgent crisis than starvation but it is still a serious problem in the developing world.**
- **Malnutrition in children often prevents normal physical and intellectual growth.**
- **Political, social, and environmental issues all play a role in poverty and hunger.**
- **Wars are one of the biggest political causes of hunger and malnutrition.**

3 Nutrition & Poverty in the Developing World

In many nations of the developed world, food is thrown away every day. Meanwhile, millions of people are going hungry. In the developing nations, people are literally starving.

The statistics are overwhelming. If you think about them, realizing that each number refers to human lives just like yours, you will get an idea how enormous this problem really is:

- Every year 15 million children in the developing nations die of hunger.

- The World Health Organization (WHO) estimates that one-third of the world is well-fed, one-third is under-fed, and one-third is starving. Well-fed people are found around the world, as are under-fed people, but almost all starving people are found in the developing world.

- Over 4 million in the developing world will die this year from starvation and malnourishment.

Economic Costs of Diet Related Chromic Disease, China and Sri Lanka

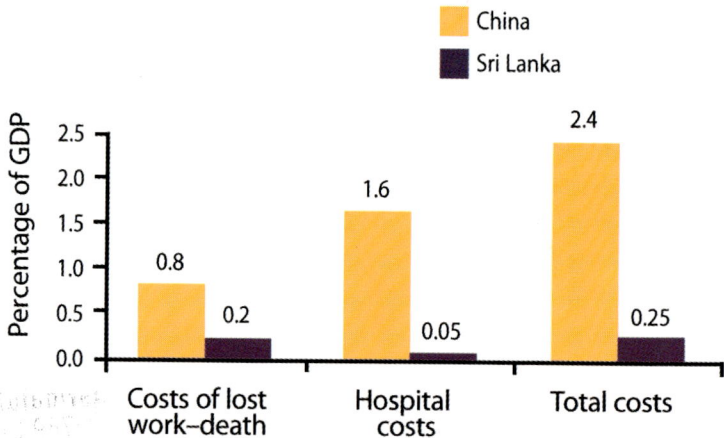

- The Indian subcontinent has nearly half the world's hungry people. Africa and the rest of Asia together have approximately 40 percent, and the remaining hungry people are found in Latin America and other parts of the world.

- Half of all children under five years of age in South Asia and one third of those in sub-Saharan Africa are malnourished. They may consume enough calories (usually in the form of cheap carbohydrates such as rice and wheat), but they do not have enough protein and vitamins in their diet. This lack of nutrients interferes with their development and health.

- Every 3.6 seconds someone in the developing world dies of hunger. That means that

Ask the Doctor

Q: I've heard that fast food isn't just bad for you because it has so many fat calories but that it's also bad for our planet. I don't understand how that could be.

Much of the meat in the hamburgers sold by fast food chains comes from cows raised in South America. This means that acres of land there go toward feeding hungry North Americans (and others around the world, since fast food is a growing trend)—rather than being used for farmland that could help feed local populations who are meanwhile living in poverty.

Chronic Disease and Childhood Malnutrition
China and Sri Lanka

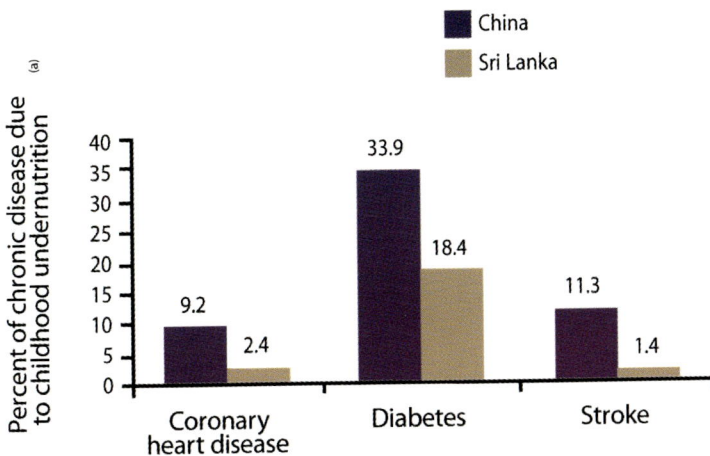

Legend: China, Sri Lanka

Percent of chronic disease due to childhood undernutrition [a]

- Coronary heart disease: China 9.2, Sri Lanka 2.4
- Diabetes: China 33.9, Sri Lanka 18.4
- Stroke: China 11.3, Sri Lanka 1.4

[a] Low birth weight and stunting

Did You Know?

In the United Kingdom, 30–40% of all food is never eaten; in the last decade the amount of food British people threw into the bin went up by 15%; and overall, £20 billion (approximately $38 billion US dollars) worth of food is thrown away, every year. Meanwhile, in the United States, 40–50% of all food ready for harvest never gets eaten.

while you read this sentence, someone died because they didn't have enough to eat.

• About 800 million people in the world suffer from hunger and malnutrition, which is around 100 times as many as those who actually die from it each year.

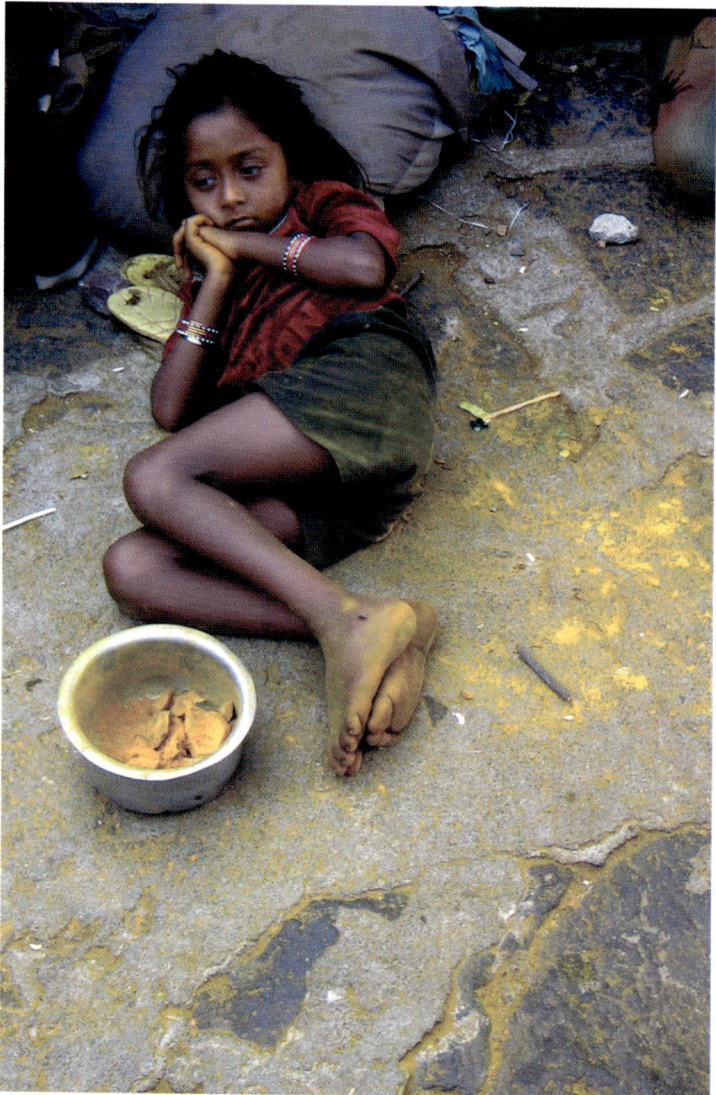

Many children in India live in extreme poverty. This child helps support her family by begging in the street.

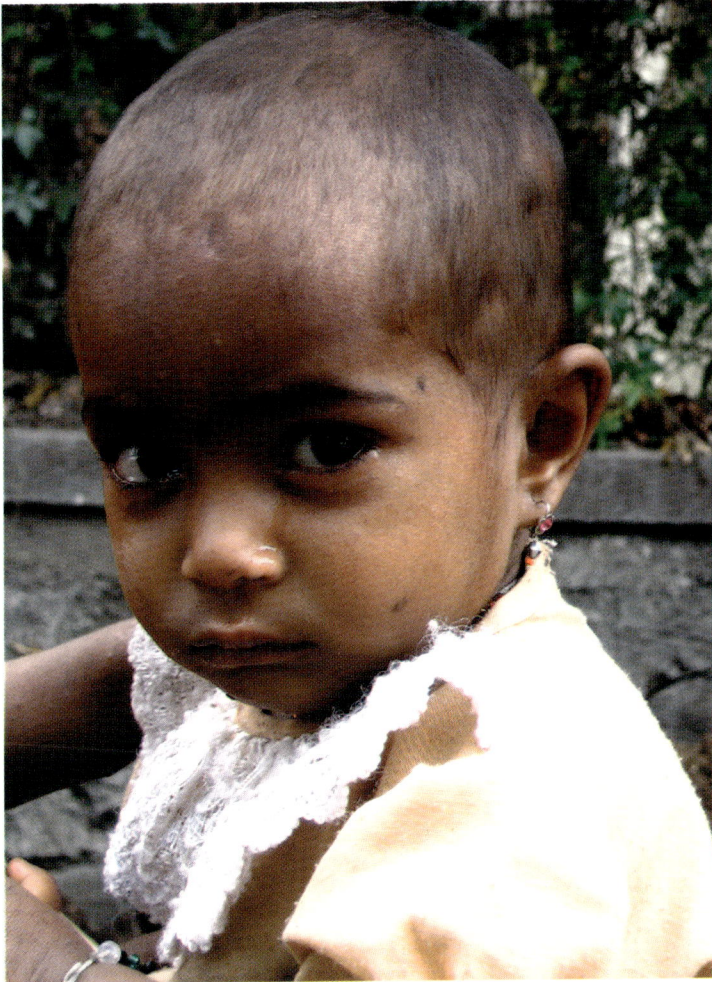

A child who grows up without all the vitamins, protein, and minerals she needs will have her entire life shaped by the malnutrition she experienced as a child.

Starvation is a more urgent crisis than malnourishment, but not eating enough nutrients to maintain good health can also lead to serious problems. Children who do not grow up eating the right kinds of food often have impaired mental and physical development; as adults, this may contribute to their not being able to earn a living, which will in turn mean that their children are more apt grow up in poverty without adequate diets. It's a terrible cycle that feeds itself generation after generation.

When a population is missing just one important nutrient from its diet, the consequences can be severe. In

Using Land in Nonproductive Ways

When farmland is used in nonproductive or even destructive ways, the overall costs to society contribute to poverty.

Examples of such land use include:

- the tobacco industry
- tea and coffee plantations
- floriculture that sells flowers in the wealthier countries
- some dam projects
- sugarcane growing for sugar exports
- fast-food industries taking land from developing nations to produce beef

many regions of the world, for example, many people do not consume enough iodine. (See chapter 1 to read why this mineral is so important.) Most developed countries add iodine to table salt, but in the developing nations of the world, this is not always in the case. Even though some nations (for instance, India) are setting up salt iodization programs, poor people are still more apt to buy non-iodized salt, which is cheaper. Producers of salt need constant encouragement to keep adding iodine to their product—and the public needs to be continually educated about the benefits of using iodized salt in their cooking.

The Link Between Poverty & Hunger

Poverty is the major cause of malnutrition and hunger. This means that when people say they want to solve the problem of world hunger, they need to realize this means the world must confront poverty. Hunger cannot be conquered unless poverty is, because the causes of hunger are related to the causes of poverty. Better growing methods for crops, improved food **distribution**, and all the charitable efforts in the world will never solve the world's nutrition issues until the root causes of poverty are faced and overcome as well.

A long list of world problems built the link between poverty and hunger. These problems are not the fault of

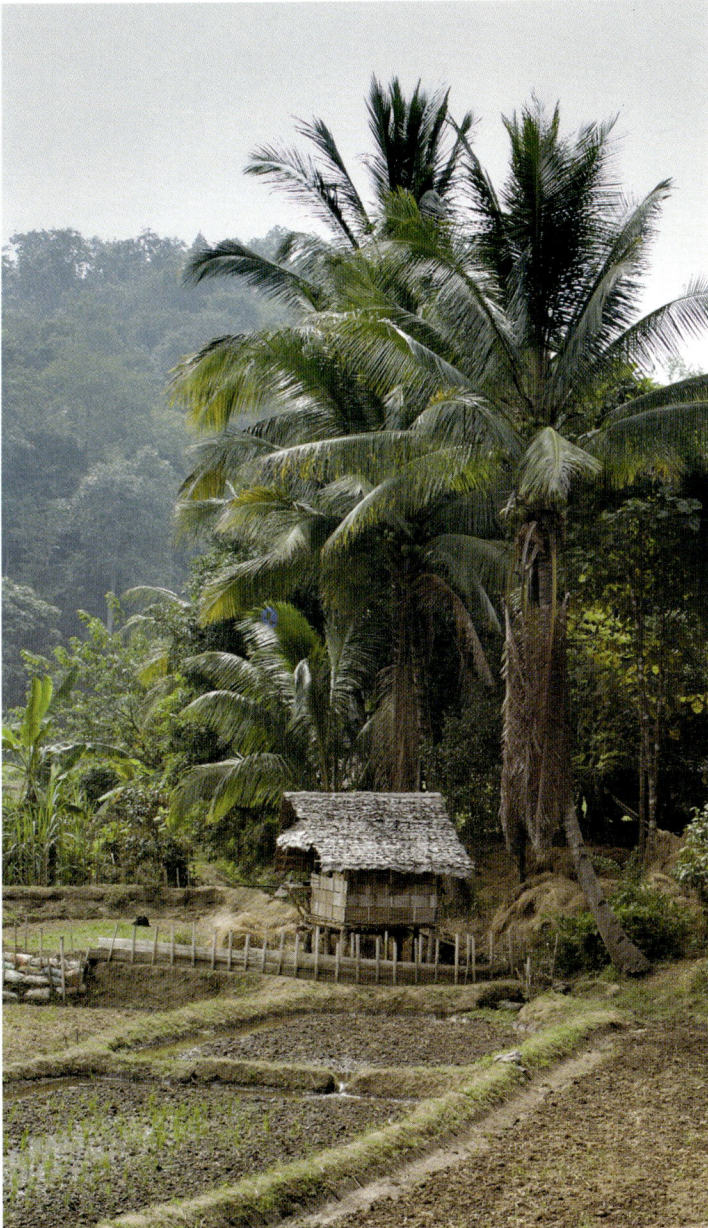

Many people in rural Thailand are subsistence farmers; they grow just enough food for themselves and their families, not enough to help feed the rest of the country. Meanwhile, in the United States, farmers sometimes throw away the extra food they grow.

the developing nations; many of them are the result of actions taken by the developed countries of the world. Environmental factors are at the root of others. The list includes:

- lack of land rights and ownership in many parts of the developing world
- using land for uses other than food production
- an increasing emphasis on farming that ships foods to other countries rather than feeding local populations

A tea plantation in Malaysia covers acres of land that could be used for growing food.

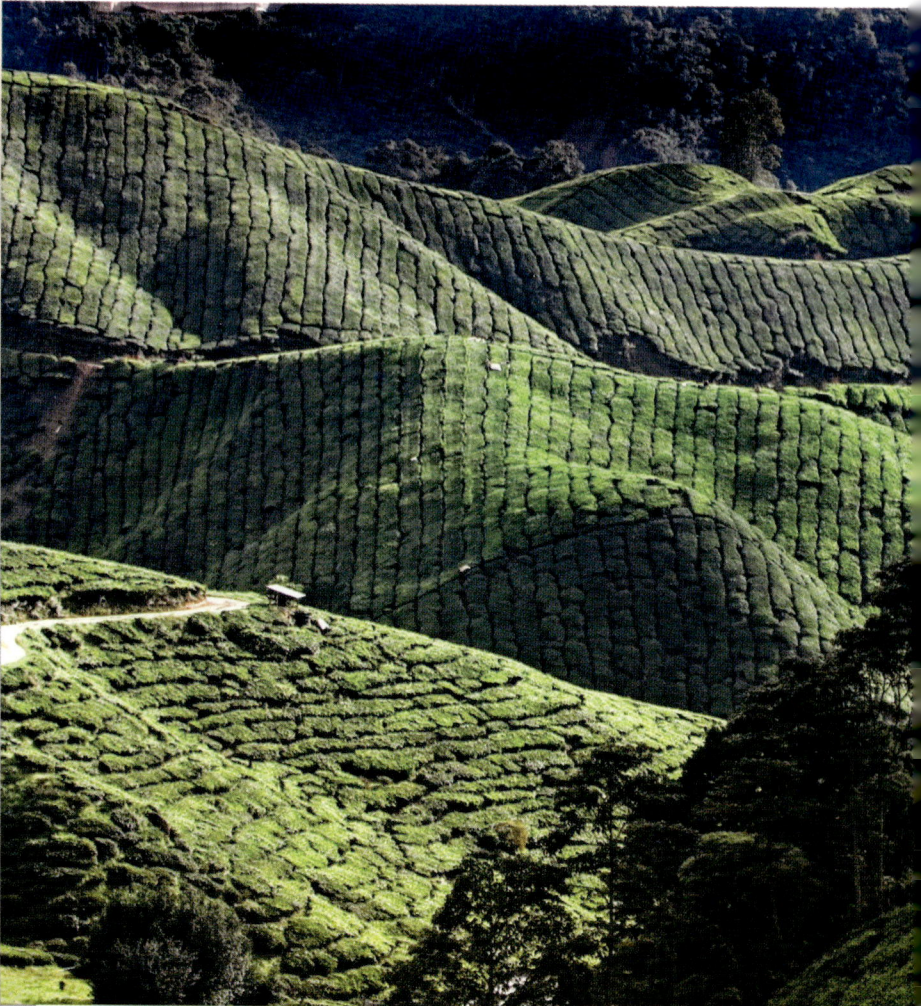

- **inefficient** farming practices
- war
- **famine**
- **drought**
- over-fishing
- poor **crop yield**
- lack of **democracy** and **human rights**

Clearly, the items on this list are interwoven. Inefficient farming techniques and drought contribute to poor

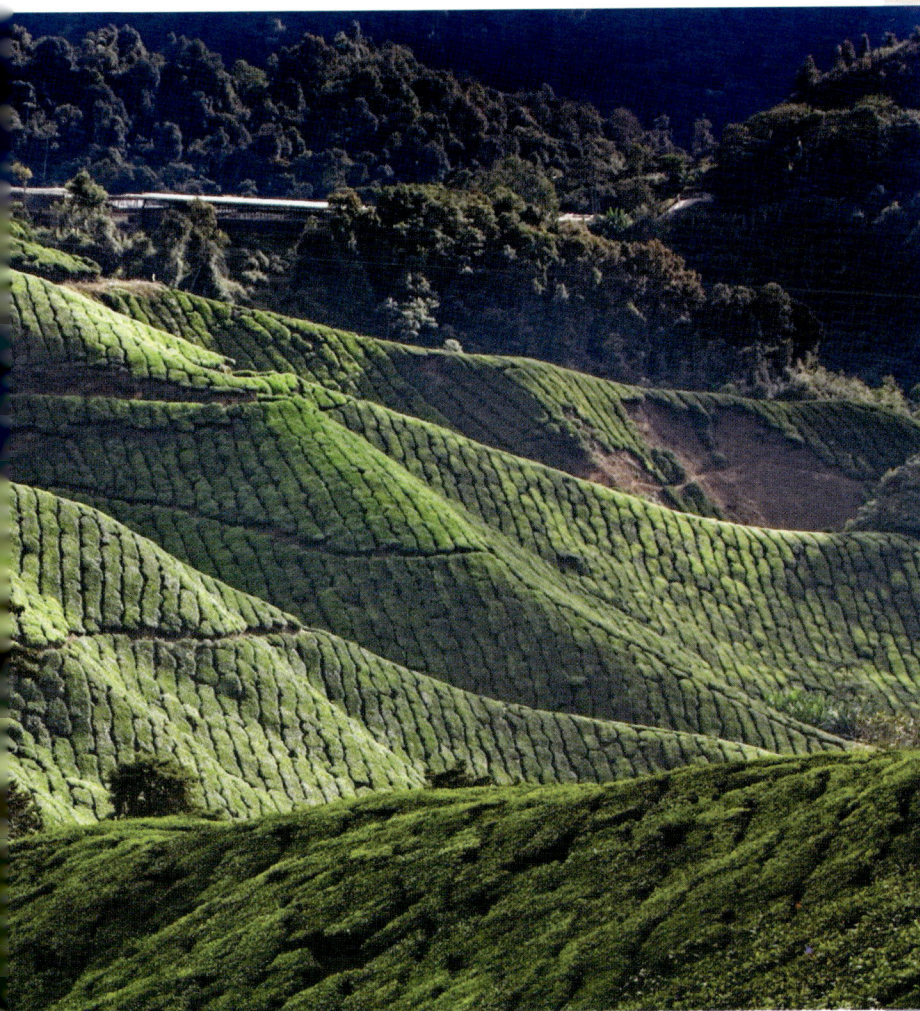

Real People

People worldwide are coping [with the current food crisis] in different ways. For the 1 billion living on less than a dollar a day, it is a matter of survival. In a mud hut on the Sahara's edge, Manthita Sou, a 43-year-old widow in the Mauritanian desert village of Maghleg, is confronting wheat prices that are up 67 percent on local markets in the past year. Her solution: stop eating bread. Instead, she has downgraded to cheaper foods, such as sorghum, a dark grain widely consumed by the world's poorest people. But sorghum has jumped 20 percent in the past 12 months. Living on the 50 cents a day she earns weaving textiles to support a family of three, her answer has been to cut out breakfast, drink tea for lunch and ration a small serving of soupy sorghum meal for family dinners. "I don't know how long we can survive like this," she said.

(Source: Anthony Faiola, "The New Economics of Hunger," Washington Post, April 27, 2008, www.washingtonpost.com/wp-srv/world/globalfoodcrisis/)

crop yields; poor crop yields and wars both contribute to famines. It's nearly impossible to untangle these issues. Ultimately, however, experts believe that hunger is not caused by a lack of food. The reality is this: the Earth is capable of feeding all its people. Poverty—and the social and political systems that create poverty—is what gets in the way.

Wars are one of the biggest political factors that contribute to the world's hunger and poverty. People who cannot go into fields for fear they will be killed by gunshot or landmines cannot grow the food they need to live; people who have to flee their homes to escape war's violence must leave behind their farms, their food supplies, and their livelihoods. When a region has suffered a combination of factors—for example, a drought and a civil war—the crisis becomes deadly.

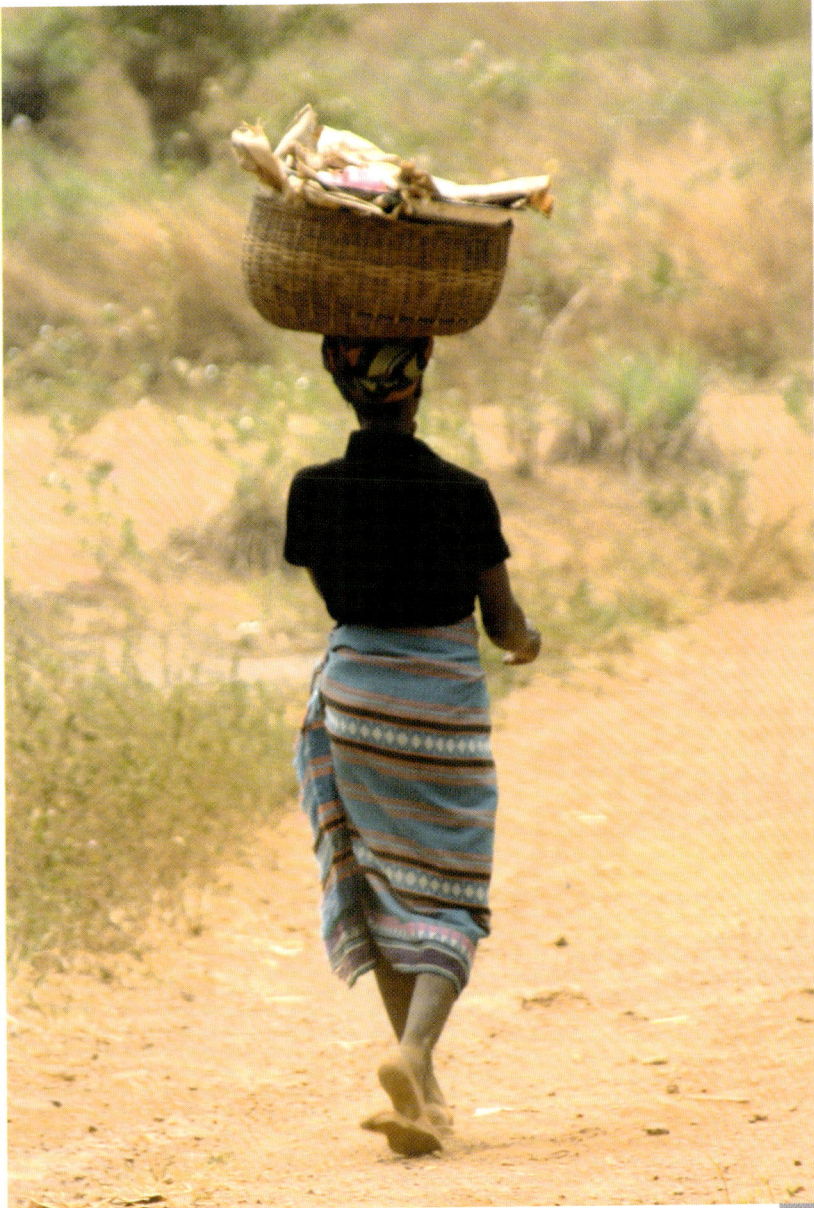

This woman is from Sierra Leone, where many families were forced to flee their homes to escape civil war.

Many African nations have faced this ongoing crisis for decades. Author Amartya Sen explains how wars and hunger have been connected in the continent's nations:

> The urgency of peace in Africa is hard to overstate. Many of the recent famines in sub-Saharan countries have been directly connected with military conflicts (for example, in Ethiopia, Sudan, Somalia, Uganda, Chad, Nigeria and Mozambique). Wars not only lead to massacres and associated horrors, they also destroy crops and other economic resources, undermine traditional patterns of livelihood, discourage economic investment, . . . and also disrupt the normal operations of trade and commerce. They also help *consoli-*

In the Sudan, civil wars have destroyed crops and ways of life, meaning that people are even more likely to be affected by poverty than they would be normally.

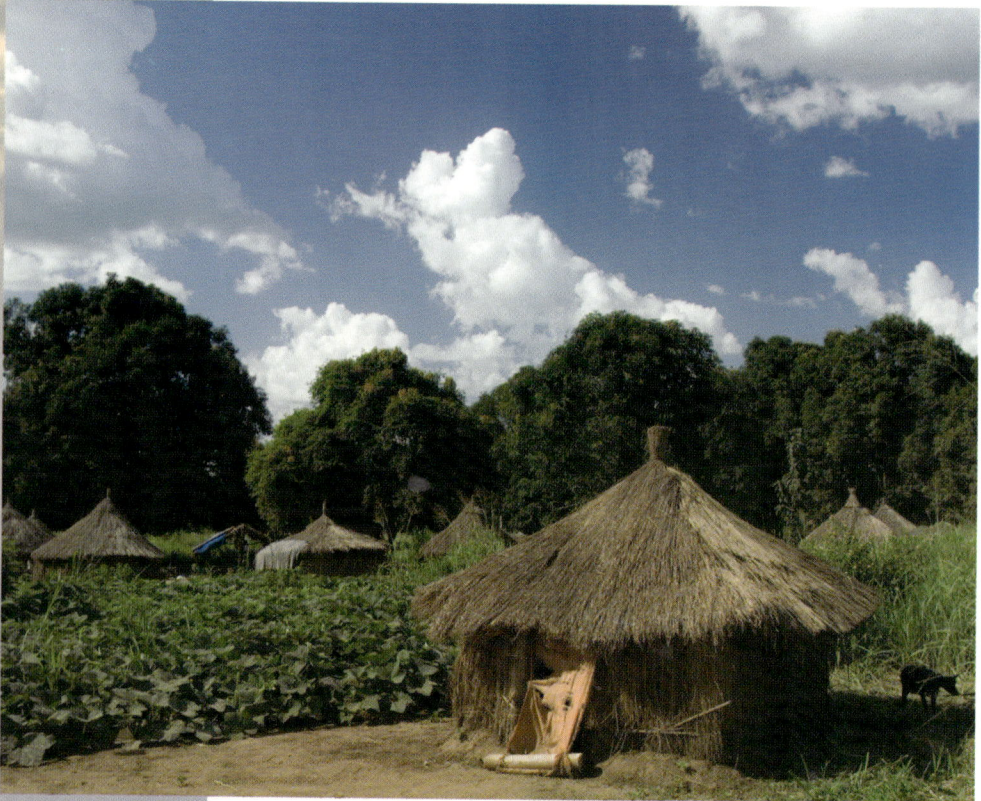

date the grip of the military on civil life and tend to disrupt civil liberties, including the freedom of the press, which . . . is an important safeguard against famines and other man-made catastrophes.

As this author mentions, democracy and human rights issues play a central role in both poverty and hunger. In political systems where only the richest members of the nation have power, the poor "do not matter," and they have no political voice to change their situation. Sen explains that "democracy and an uncensored press can spread the penalty of famines from the destitute to those in authority. There is no surer way of making the government responsive to the suffering of famine victims [than to allow democracy and a free press to flourish]."

Clearly, though, democracy and a free press alone cannot guarantee that hunger will be wiped off the Earth. After all, democratic nations also face the challenge of hunger and malnutrition.

STRAIGHT FROM THE SOURCE

(From J.W. Smith's The World's Wasted Wealth: The Political Economy of Waste, New World's Press, 1989.)

Who Controls the Land?

The often heard comment (one I once accepted as fact) that "there are too many people in the world, and overpopulation is the cause of hunger", can be compared to the same myth that expounded sixteenth-century England and revived continuously since.

Through repeated acts of enclosure the peasants were pushed off the land so that the gentry could make money raising wool for the new and highly productive power looms. They could not do this if the peasants were to retain their historic entitlement to a share of production from the land. Massive starvation was the inevitable result of this expropriation.

There were serious discussions in learned circles about overpopulation as the cause of this poverty. This was the accepted reason because a social and intellectual elite were doing the rationalizing. It was they who controlled the educational institutions which studied the problem. Naturally the final conclusions (at least those published) absolved the wealthy of any responsibility for the plight of the poor. The absurdity of suggesting that England was then overpopulated is clear when we realize that "the total population of England in the sixteenth century was less than in any one of several present-day English cities."

The hunger in underdeveloped countries today is equally tragic and absurd. Their European colonizers understood well that ownership of land gave the owner control over what society produced. The most powerful simply redistributed the valuable land titles to themselves, eradicating millennia-old traditions of common use. Since custom is a form of ownership, the shared use of land could not be permitted. If ever reestablished, this ancient practice would reduce the rights of these new owners. For this reason, much of the land went unused or underused until the owners could do so profitably. This is the pattern of land use that characterizes most Third World countries today, and it is this that generates hunger in the world.

What Do You Think?

- Why would a free press make those in power pay the "penalty of famine"?

Here's what you need to know

- Millions of people in the developed nations of the world suffer from under-nourishment and malnutrition.
- Poverty and race are often linked with hunger in the developed world.
- Obesity is also a big problem in developed nations—and obesity is also linked with poverty and malnutrition.
- "Food insecurity" is a term used to describe people in developed nations who have difficulty at least some of the time buying the food they need.

Words to Understand

Mortality rate refers to the death rate, expressed as the number of deaths per 1000 people per year.

Obesity is the state of being extremely overweight to a point where it can cause us health problems.

Economies refers to systems of exchange of goods. Most modern economies are based on money, but older and simpler communities may rely on barter systems.

4

Nutrition & Poverty in the Developed World

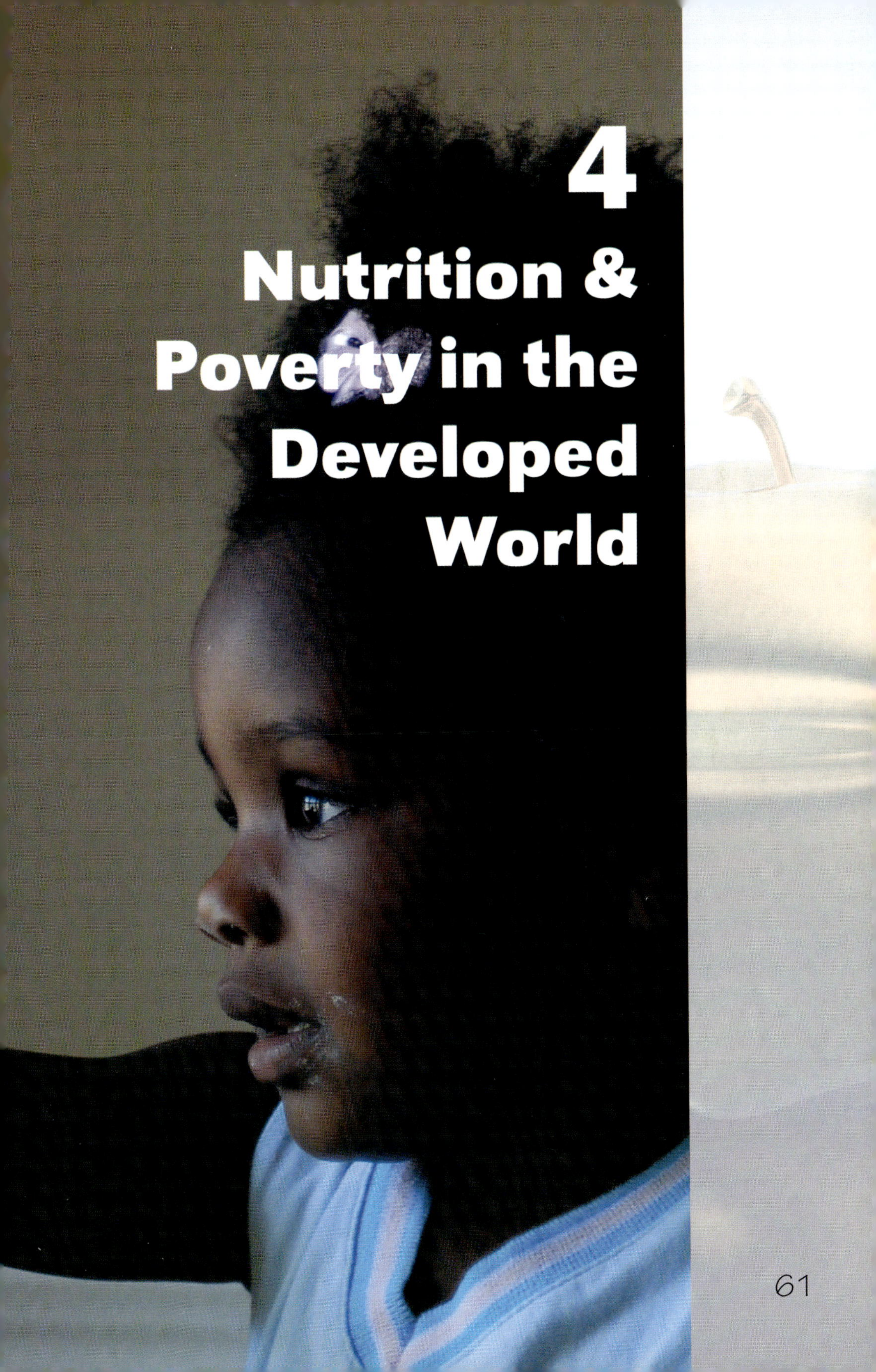

It's not only developing nations where people suffer from malnutrition and related diseases. The problem reaches into the world's developed nations as well.

Undernourishment & Malnutrition

In the United States, according to the U.S. Department of Agriculture, more than 13 million families in 2004 were unable at times to buy the food they needed. Finances were so strained for 5 million of these families that one or more of their members often went hungry. In other developed nations of the world (including the United States), 2 billion people living in poverty, mostly women, babies, and children, lack the iron, iodine, or vitamin A they need.

Race, poverty, and hunger are intertwined in the developed world. People from many minority groups are more apt to live in poverty, and in the United States, 46 percent of black American children are hungry nearly every day, while 40 percent of Latino children are hungry—compared to only 16 percent of all white children.

People who live in poverty in the developed nations have higher infant mortality rates, and this has been linked to inadequate nutrition among pregnant women.

Real People

"With all of my expenses, sometimes I have to go to bed without eating. I am used to it," a North American woman told a social worker. "I buy the medication first. I cook macaroni and put some sauce on it. No protein you know, not enough protein."

This woman feels she has no options. She has to take her medicine or she could die. So she fills up her stomach as best she can, whenever she can.

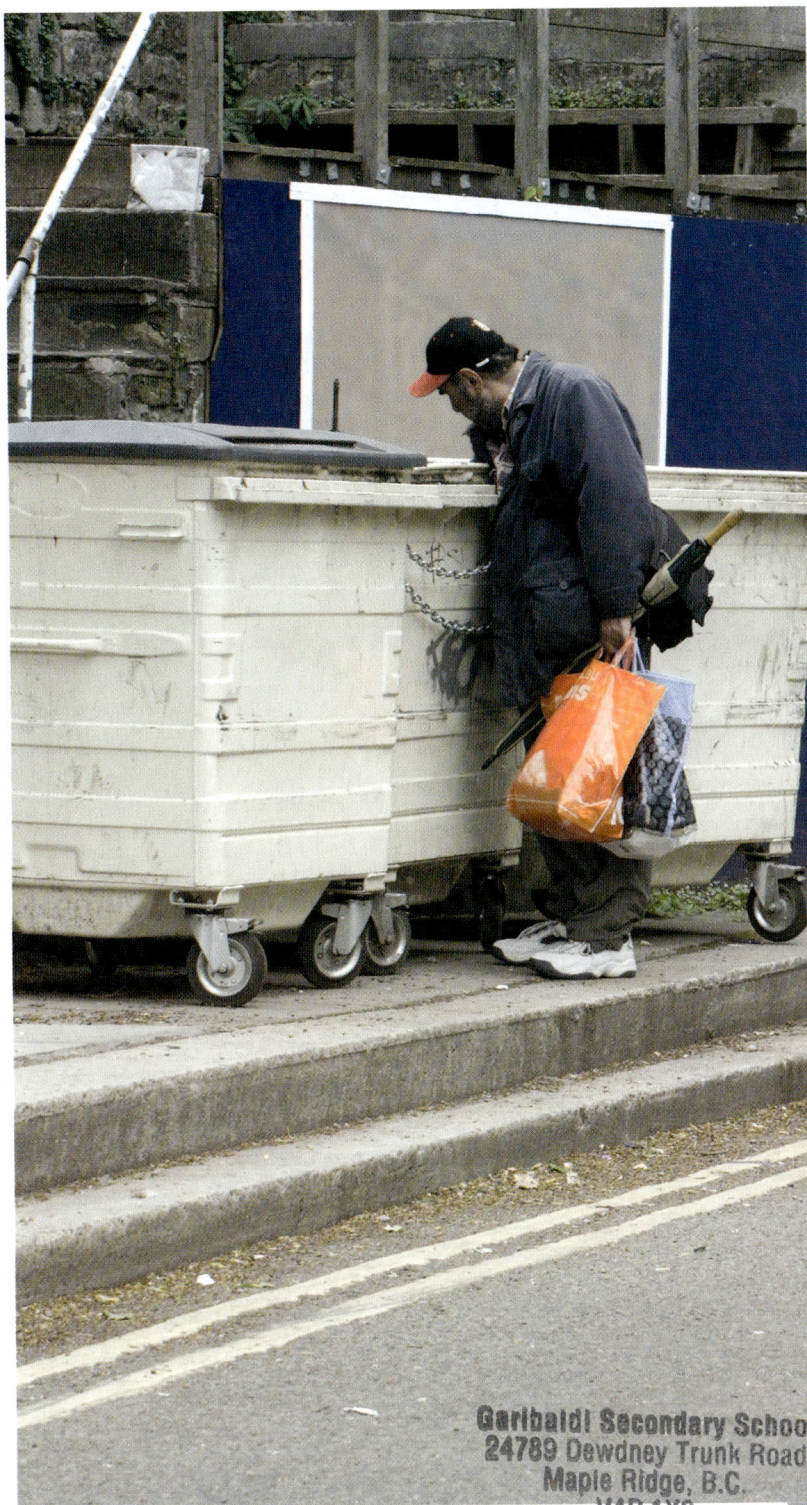

The developed nations of the world also have people living in poverty. Homelessness is a growing problem in many urban areas. For this man, a dumpster full of other people's garbage is a resource that offers food, clothing, and other goods.

The United States ranks twenty-third in infant mortality among the developed nations, and black American babies die at nearly twice the rate of white ones.

According to the United Nations, one in twelve people in the developed world is malnourished, including 160 million children under the age of five. In the United States, one out of every six elderly people have inadequate diets, and one out of eight children under the age of twelve goes to bed hungry every night. These people aren't starving to death—but they don't have the nutrition they need to be healthy.

Grocery stores in developed nations are stocked with every possible food product—but if you lack the funds to buy them, these shelves of plenty do you little good.

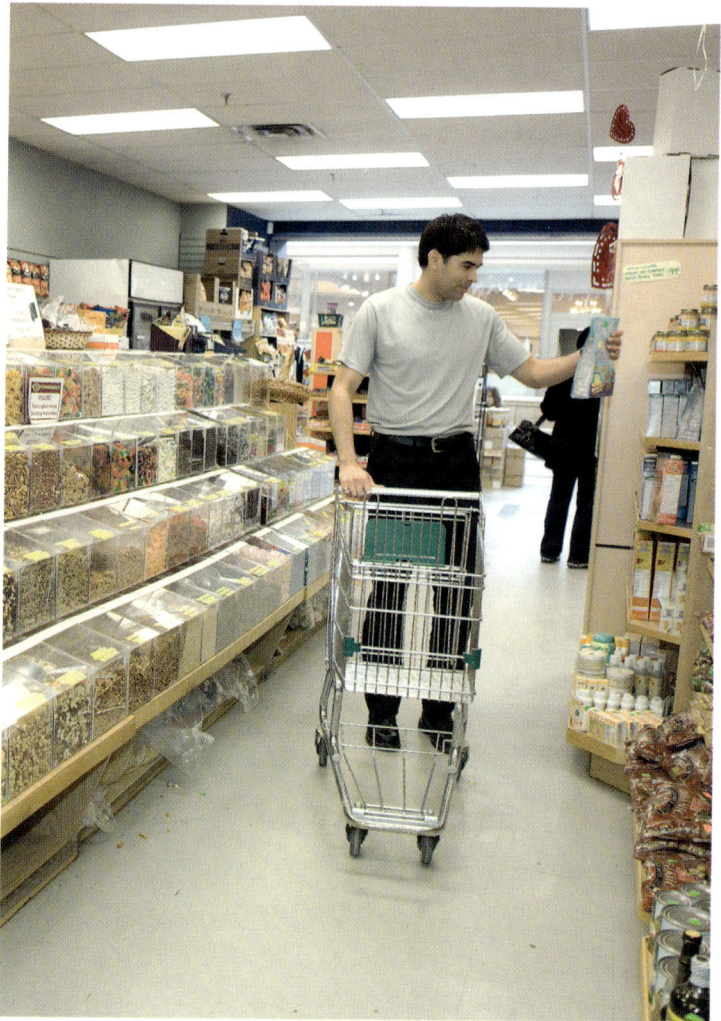

GDP loss from Reduced Adult Productivity Due to Some Forms of Undernutrition

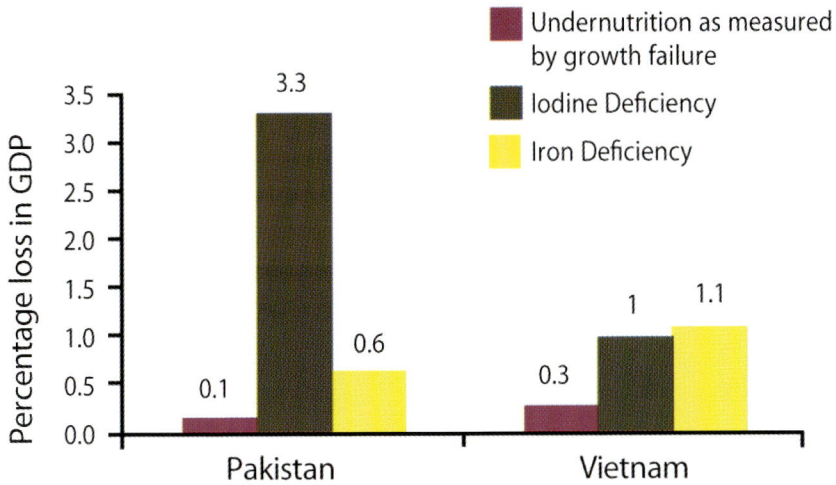

Legend:
- Undernutrition as measured by growth failure
- Iodine Deficiency
- Iron Deficiency

Percentage loss in GDP

Pakistan: 0.1, 3.3, 0.6
Vietnam: 0.3, 1, 1.1

GDP Loss Due to Iron Deficiency

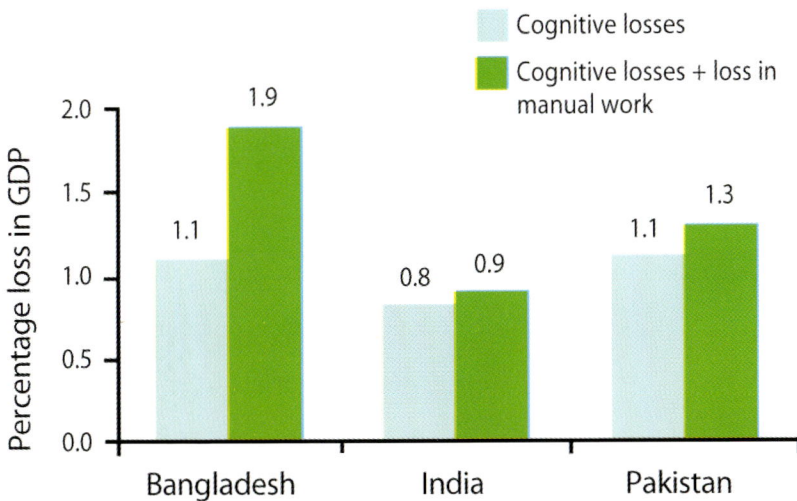

Legend:
- Cognitive losses
- Cognitive losses + loss in manual work

Percentage loss in GDP

Bangladesh: 1.1, 1.9
India: 0.8, 0.9
Pakistan: 1.1, 1.3

If you live in a developing nation, food may be more apt to come from the land than from a store. Food stores may be few and far between—and the ones that exist often have empty shelves. But in the developed countries of the world, grocery stores are in every town and city, and they're full of all kinds of foods and vitamin-supplemented products. But despite this, many children and pregnant mothers aren't getting the nutrients they need for good health. Meanwhile child and adult **obesity** is a serious concern.

Obesity

Obesity is a growing problem in the world's developed nations. People who have less money are apt to choose cheaper high-calorie foods, rather than make more expensive—and healthier—choices.

You might think that obesity is just the opposite problem from malnutrition and undernourishment. But that's not the case. Many people who are obese don't eat a balanced diet. They tend to eat calorie-dense foods (like bread, desserts, pasta, rice, potatoes, and fast food), rather than more expensive nutrient-dense foods. This means that their bodies are storing the extra calories in the form of fat,

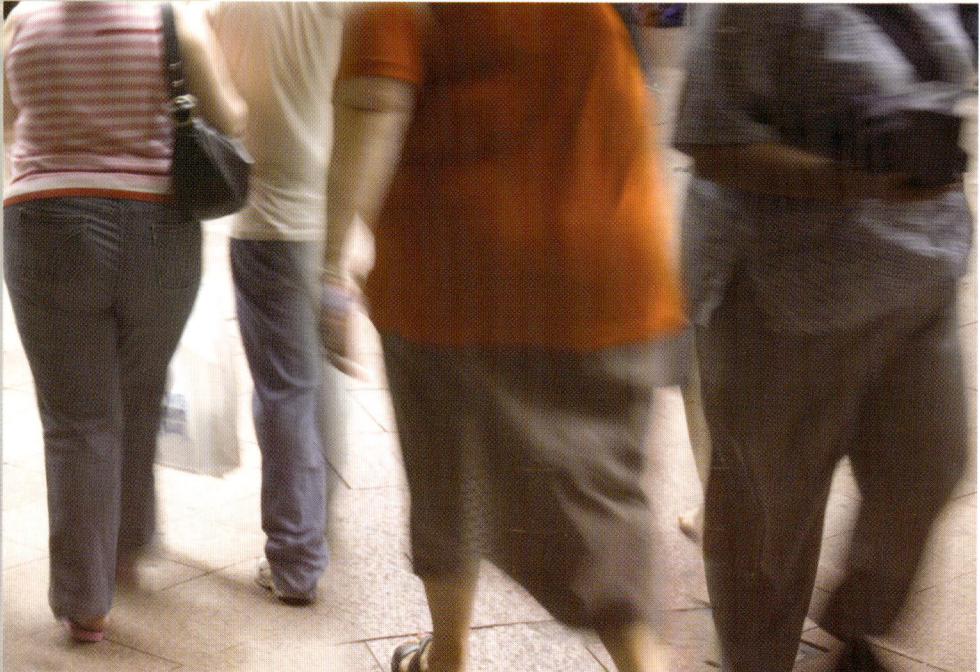

How Is Obesity Determined?

One tool doctors use to evaluate body size is body mass index (BMI). BMI is a mathematical formula that uses weight and height to determine whether someone's body is a healthy size. The formula is as follows:

[Weight in pounds ÷ (Height in inches x Height in inches)] x 703 = BMI
[weight in kilograms ÷ (Height in meters x Height in meters)] = BMI

A BMI that is:
Below 18.5 = Underweight
18.5 – 24.9 = Normal
25.0 – 29.9 = Overweight
30.0 and Above = Obese

Example for a person who weighs 132 pounds and is five-feet, four-inches (64 inches) tall:
[132 pounds ÷ (64 inches x 64 inches)] x 703 = 22.66 (a normal weight)

BMI is not always an accurate measure of health. Muscle tissue is much denser and heavier than fat tissue. Since BMI only measures height and weight, an extremely muscular and fit person could have the same BMI as an unfit person who has a large amount of fat. For this reason, a better measure of obesity is body fat percentage—the amount of your body's tissue that is made of fat. Doctors, nutritionists, and fitness experts use tools to measure different areas of the body. These measurements yield one's body fat percentage.

while all the while they're not getting the nutrients they need for good health.

Poverty often plays a role in this. Calorie-dense foods tend to be cheaper than nutrient-dense ones. They fill you up without costing a lot of money. Unfortunately, they also make you fat without providing the vitamins, minerals, and protein you need for good health. Frozen and canned foods are also less expensive than fresh foods—but the processing that takes place during freezing and canning breaks down a food's structure, removing nutrients.

Did You Know?

Almost two-thirds—64.5 percent—of all Americans are overweight or obese. That's 127 million people.

Did You Know?

In many poor, rural American communities, families often have no choice but to use the emergency room for their health care needs. This is very expensive, but jobs and income depend on health—and transportation. So if the family car needs repair, a family will have no choice but to again reduce food intake to get the car back on the road in order to go to work.

Obesity risk factors and poverty are often linked. The Food Research and Action Center lists the following factors that contribute to this connection:

Low-income neighborhoods are underserved by full-service supermarkets.

- Low-income neighborhoods frequently lack full-service grocery stores and farmers' markets where residents can buy fruits, vegetables, whole grains, and low-fat dairy products. Instead, residents often are limited to shopping at small neighborhood convenience stores, where fresh produce and low-fat food items are limited, if available at all.

When available, healthy food is more expensive.

- The price of healthy foods is also a factor for many low-income households—healthy foods often are

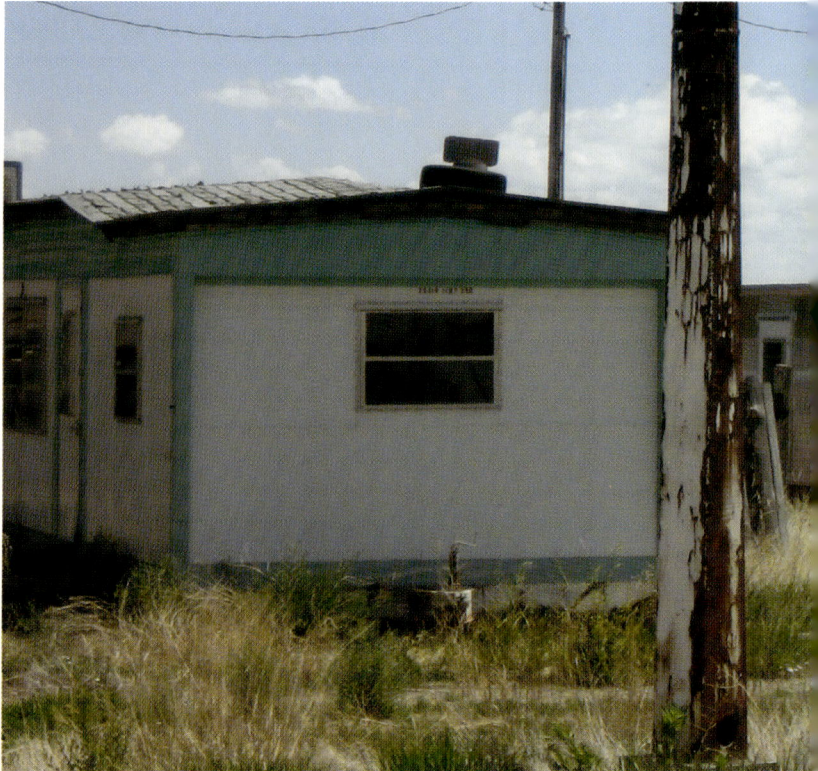

significantly more expensive, when they are available.

• Low-income families that are trying to stretch their dollars may be forced to buy cheaper, higher calorie foods in order to make their food budgets last.

There are few opportunities for physical activity in neighborhoods and schools.

• Low-income neighborhoods often have few safe or attractive places to play or be physically active. Open space—good parks, sidewalks, and fields—is at a minimum, and recreational facilities often are inadequate.

• High rates of crime or fear of crime make parents reluctant to permit children to play and be physically active outdoors. After-school and summertime recreational activities and sports are also typically less available to low-income children.

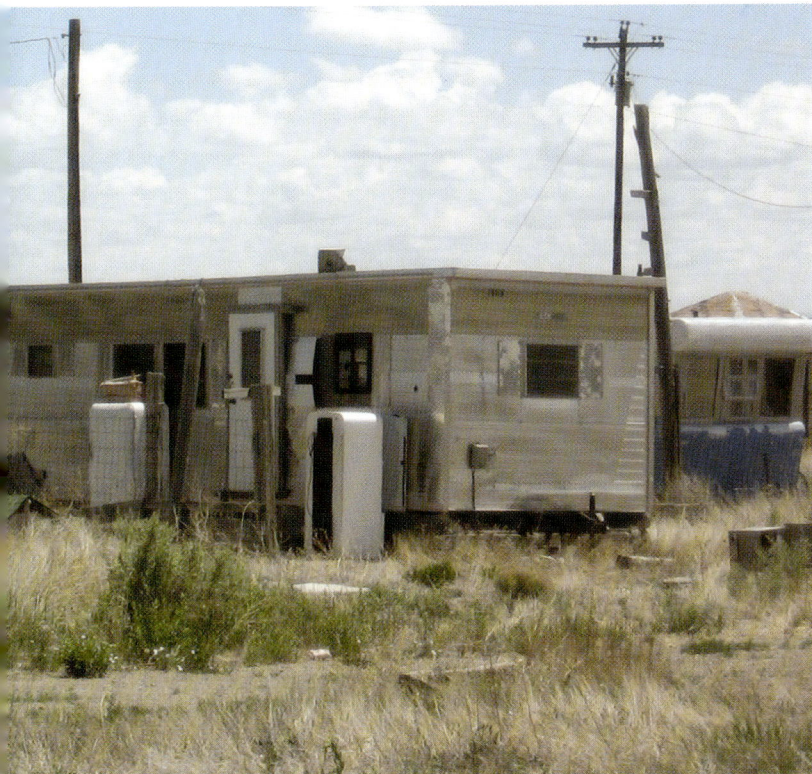

A rural trailer park in the U.S. state of New Mexico shows another version of poverty. The people who live here often experience food insecurity.

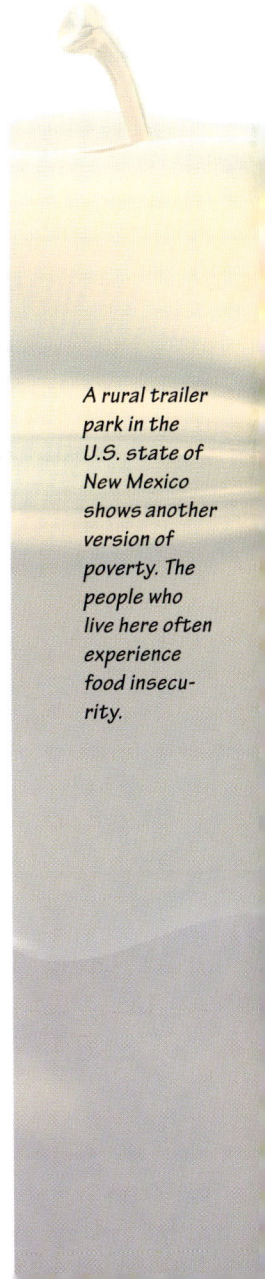

• School districts in low-income neighborhoods are frequently underfunded, making cutbacks in physical education more likely. This also puts pressure on schools to supplement their funds by permitting the sale of less healthy foods in competition with the school breakfast and lunch programs.

High levels of stress and limited access to health care can contribute to weight gain.

• Hunger may be a stressor that results in disordered eating, reduced physical activity, and depression, all of which may be related to weight gain. And hunger and/or poverty may also cause a stress response that is hormonal, and contributes to obesity.

Food Insecurity

Some experts use the term "food insecure" to refer to people who have difficulty at least some of the time buying the food they need. They go hungry because of unexpected circumstances: car repairs, an emergency visit to the hospital, a sudden loss of a job. When faced with events like these, families have to make a tradeoff between food and other expenses.

For people who normally live above the poverty line, a single crisis can push them over the edge into poverty. This means that groceries are probably the first place they will cut their expenses. Food is usually purchased with cash, and if you don't have it, you can't buy food. More grocery stores accept credit cards now, but many people in these circumstances don't have "plastic"—and if they do, the cards become rapidly overdrawn in the midst of a financial crisis.

Ask the Doctor

I weigh 140 pounds and I'm five-foot-five. Am I obese?

No, you're not. In fact, you're not even overweight. When doctors use the words "overweight" and "obese," they're not referring to having an extra few pounds of body weight. Instead they're referring to a medical condition where a person has so much extra body weight that it affects health. North American culture tends to put too much value on thin bodies, when people can be perfectly healthy (and look just fine as well) with a little extra weight. Use the formula for determining BMI to give yourself a better idea of what you should weigh—but keep in mind that other factors can play a role in weight besides fat. If you're still concerned, ask your doctor's advice.

According to the United Nations, the ability to obtain enough food for an active, healthy life is one of the most basic of human rights. Food-insecure households cannot achieve this most basic level of well-being. When nations that have otherwise successful economies have such high levels of undernourishment and malnutrition, something is very wrong. These people, as well as the people who live in crisis-level hunger situations in the world's developing nations, deserve the world's help.

STRAIGHT FROM THE SOURCE

(From Food Research and Action Center fact sheet, www.frac. org/pdf/factsheet_foodcosts_apr08.pdf)

The Impact of Rising Food Costs on Low-Income Americans

All Americans are starting to feel the pinch of food costs that suddenly have begun rising more rapidly, on top of rising energy, housing, and health costs. The higher cost of food is falling especially hard on low-income families—the people already stretching limited budgets to the utmost. In a crunch, for many households food costs are the main area where they choose to cut back on spending, albeit at a price to their health. Bills for rent or mortgage, child care and transportation to work must be paid, as well as heating costs and the water bill. Cutting back on groceries, as painful as it may be, can seem like the only choice to make.

FACTS AT YOUR FINGERTIPS:

- According to the Department of Labor, the cost of food at home rose 4.7 percent from March 2007–March 2008.

- Some food items experienced a double-digit increase in price during the same time period, including:

   —Milk increased by 13.3 percent.

   —Eggs increased by 29.9 percent.

   —Cheese increased by 12.5 percent.

   —Bread increased by 14.7 percent.

- The price of a market basket of basics on which low-income people rely rose even faster. From February 2007 to February 2008, the cost of the

"Thrifty Food Plan" rose by 6.3 percent. The Thrifty Food Plan is the government's basis for Food Stamp allotments—it represents the least expensive basket of food the government prices (and recommends only for short-term use). Studies show that most families cannot actually obtain a healthy diet with this level of spending, but it is what many low-income families are relegated to, at best.

- Because some parts of the food stamp benefit computation are not indexed for inflation, and those that are indexed are changed only once a year (in October), faster food inflation especially harms people on food stamps.

What Do You Think?

- What expenses does this document indicate take priority over food in many low-income American households?

- If you were to fill a grocery basket full of the most basic foods you and your family would need to get by for a week, what would you put in the basket? How much do you think it would cost?

- How does inflation have an impact on nutrition?

Find Out More

Go to these Web sites to get more information on nutrition and poverty in the developed world:

Homelessness
www.faqs.org/nutrition/Hea-Irr/Homelessness.html

Hunger in a Land of Plenty
www.indiancountry.com/content.cfm?id=1096417186

Here's what you need to know

- **The United Nations is leading the world's battle against malnutrition and poverty.**
- **The UN's Millennium Development Goals give the world 8 important goals to achieve by 2015 in order to end poverty.**
- **Many famous people and charities have joined the fight against hunger and poverty.**
- **Bono from the rock group U2 is one of the leading stars who is fighting hunger and poverty.**
- **NGOs—non-governmental organizations—are people who have joined together to fight a particular cause.**
- **NGOs have led the battle against hunger and poverty, and are working with the United Nations to do still more.**

Words to Understand

Momentum is the speed of movement, the push that builds to continue going forward once something is set in motion.

Something or someone who is **influential** has the ability to bring about change.

Socially has to do with human interactions.

Economically has to do with money and finances.

Politically has to do with governments.

Activism is when people take action to bring about change.

Eradicate means to do away with something completely.

A **grassroots** movement has ordinary people getting involved to bring about change.

5
What Is the World Doing?

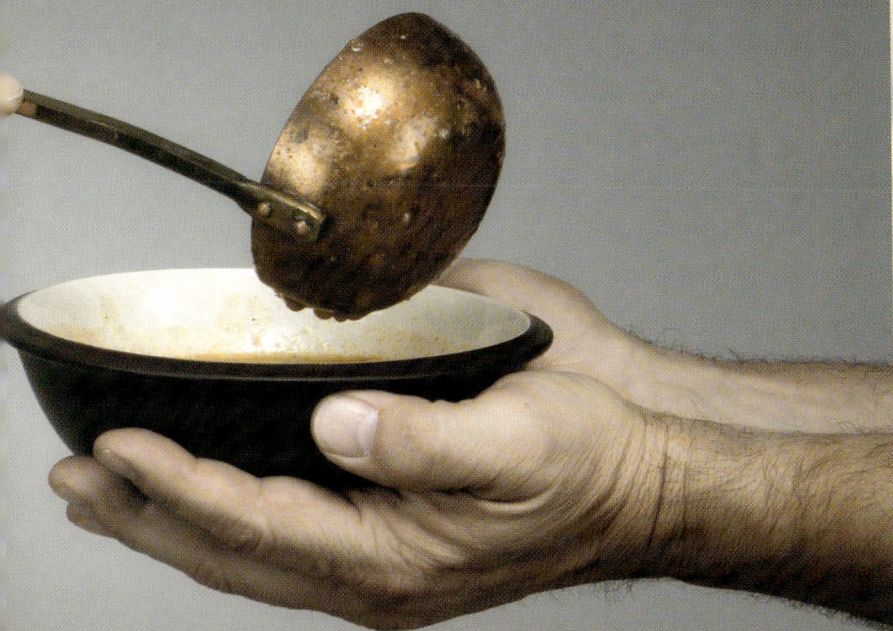

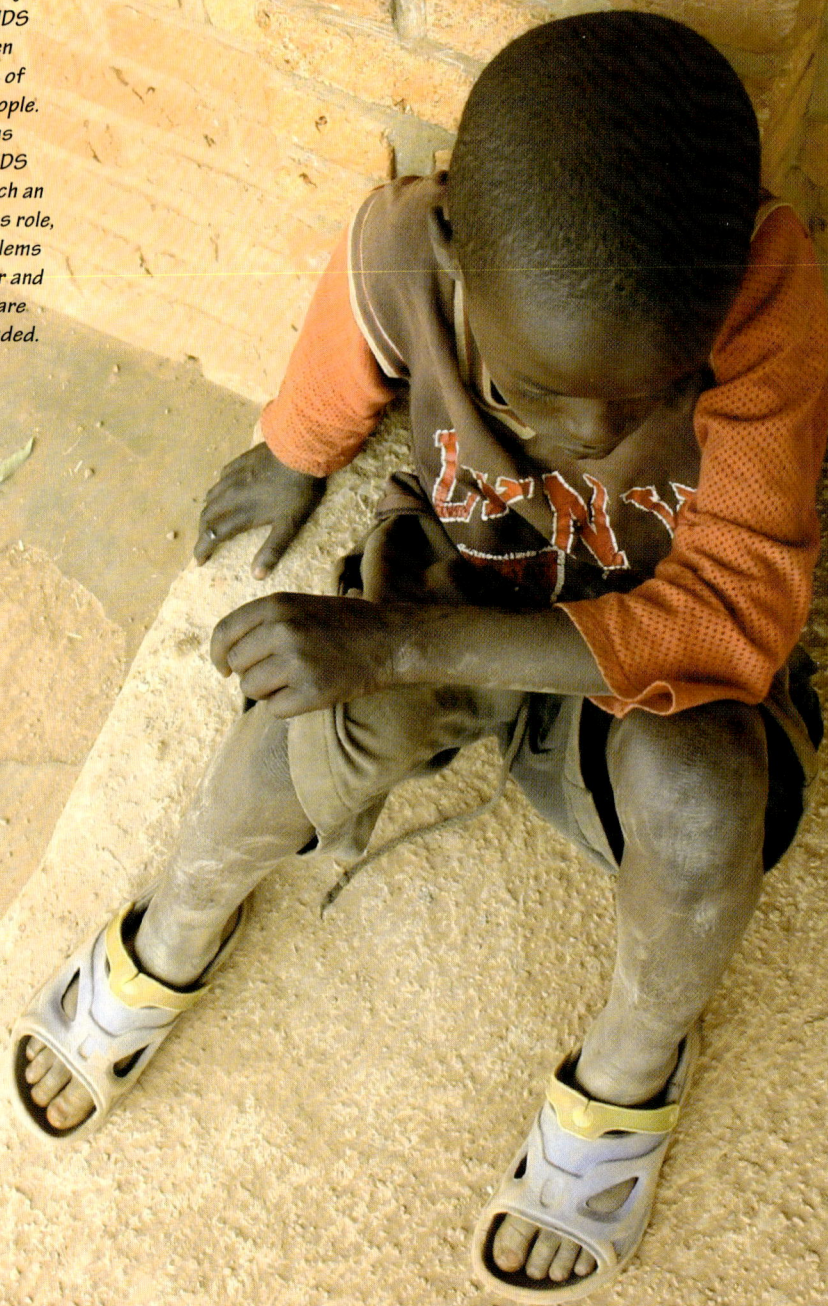

This child lives in an African community where AIDS has taken the lives of many people. In nations where AIDS plays such an enormous role, the problems of hunger and poverty are compounded.

Change seldom comes quickly, but it does come. If you learn about some of the great triumphs of human history—the end of slavery in the Western world, for example, or the right to vote for women and minorities—you'll realize that none of these changes happened overnight. Most of the time, they started out with just a few brave people willing to speak out on behalf of what was right. Those people probably felt sometimes as though the problem was just too big to tackle; they must have wondered if they were wasting their time trying to change something so big, so deeply rooted that they didn't have a chance of making a difference. But those few voices were the beginning. Gradually, more and more people listened to them, and more voices joined the call for justice. The movement gained momentum. Injustice that had once been invisible to most people became so obvious that it could no longer be ignored. Eventually, so many people spoke out so loudly that government leaders listened. New laws were passed. Little by little, the world changed.

That's what needs to happen with malnutrition and hunger. It's easy to look at the size of the problem and feel discouraged. But the same human beings who created the societies where poverty and hunger cast their shadows also have great power to do good. If you look around, you'll see that the work has already begun.

The United Nations

In September 2000, 189 of the world's nations met for the Millennium Summit. There the leaders agreed to work together to reduce poverty and improve lives. To achieve this, they issued the eight Millennium Development Goals:

1. Eradicate extreme poverty and hunger.
2. Achieve universal primary education.
3. Promote gender equality and empower women.
4. Reduce child mortality.
5. Improve maternal health.

Did You Know?

Europe's cows receive $2 a day in subsidies, more than the income of half the world's population

Did You Know?

Around the world, 115 million children are not in school; 56 percent of them are girls and 94 percent of them live in developing countries. Only 37 of 155 developing countries have achieved universal primary school completion. As a result, 133 million young people cannot read or write.

6. Combat HIV/AIDS, malaria, and other diseases.
7. Ensure environmental sustainability.
8. Develop a global partnership for development.

The United Nations' target for achieving these goals is 2015. It's an ambitious project, but Former United Nations Secretary-General Kofi A. Annan believes that together the world can achieve its goals if they make them a priority. He said:

> We will have time to reach the Millennium Development Goals—worldwide and in most, or even all, individual countries—but only if we break with business as usual. We cannot win overnight. Success will require sustained action across the entire decade between now and the deadline. It takes time to train the teachers, nurses and engineers; to build the roads, schools and hospitals; to grow the small and large businesses able to create the jobs and income needed. So we must start now. And we must more than double global development assistance over the next few years. Nothing less will help to achieve the Goals.

What does all this really mean? It means that the United Nations works with businesses, charities, other non-governmental agencies (NGOs), and private citizens to unite and coordinate many kinds of efforts to achieve the "Millennium Promise."

People Making a Difference

People all over the world are joining the fight to end hunger and poverty. Most of them have names you've probably never heard—but many of them are famous people who use their position to bring more attention to the cause they've taken on. From hip-hop artists to fashion models, movie stars to talk show hosts, more and more people are

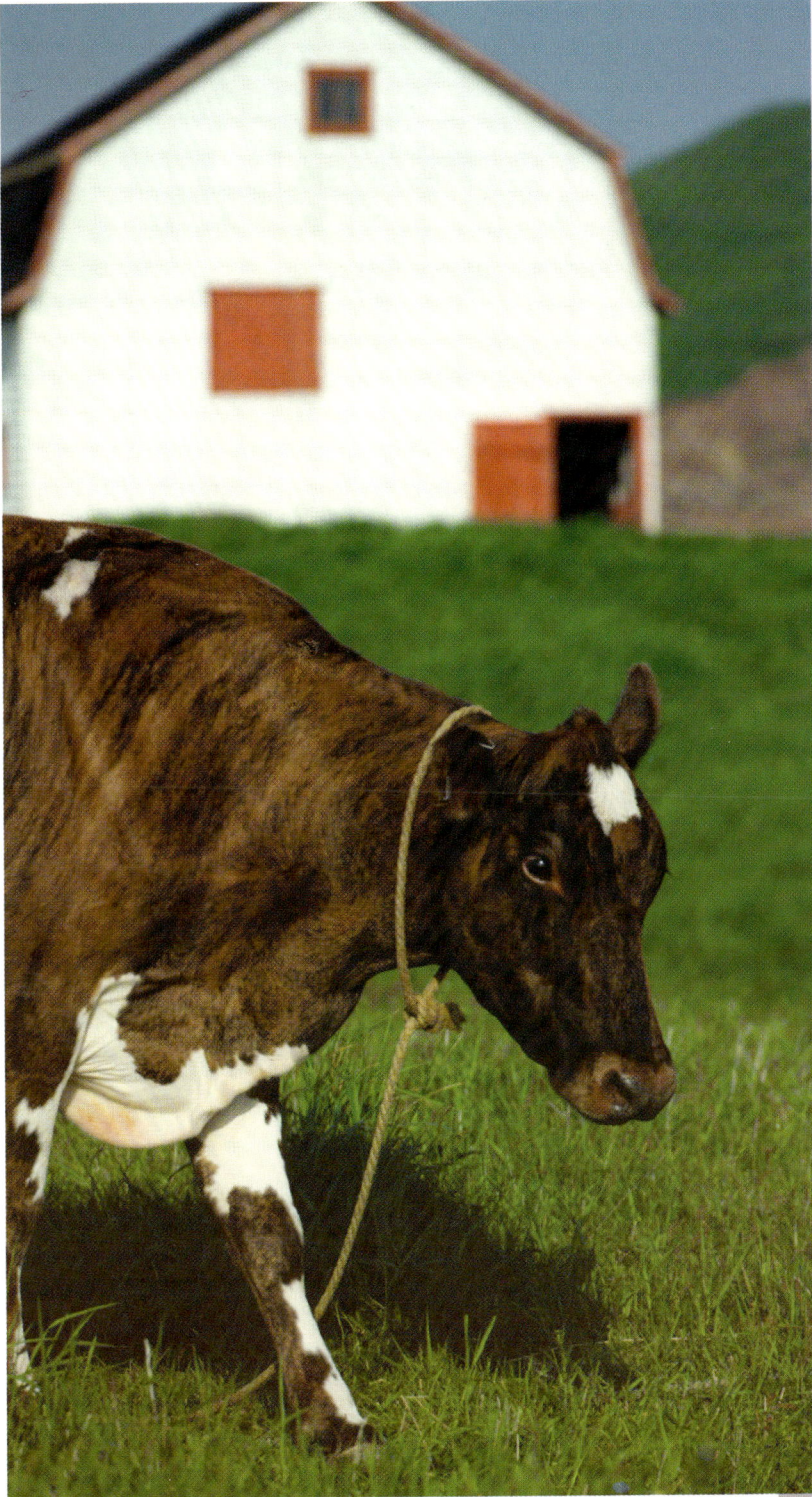

Europe's cows are fed better than many human beings are who live in poverty.

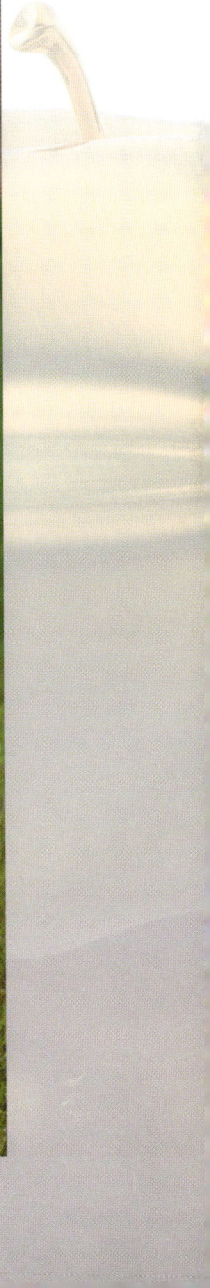

Bono is one of the people who is working to stop poverty around the world. He has been nominated for three Nobel Peace Prizes for his efforts!

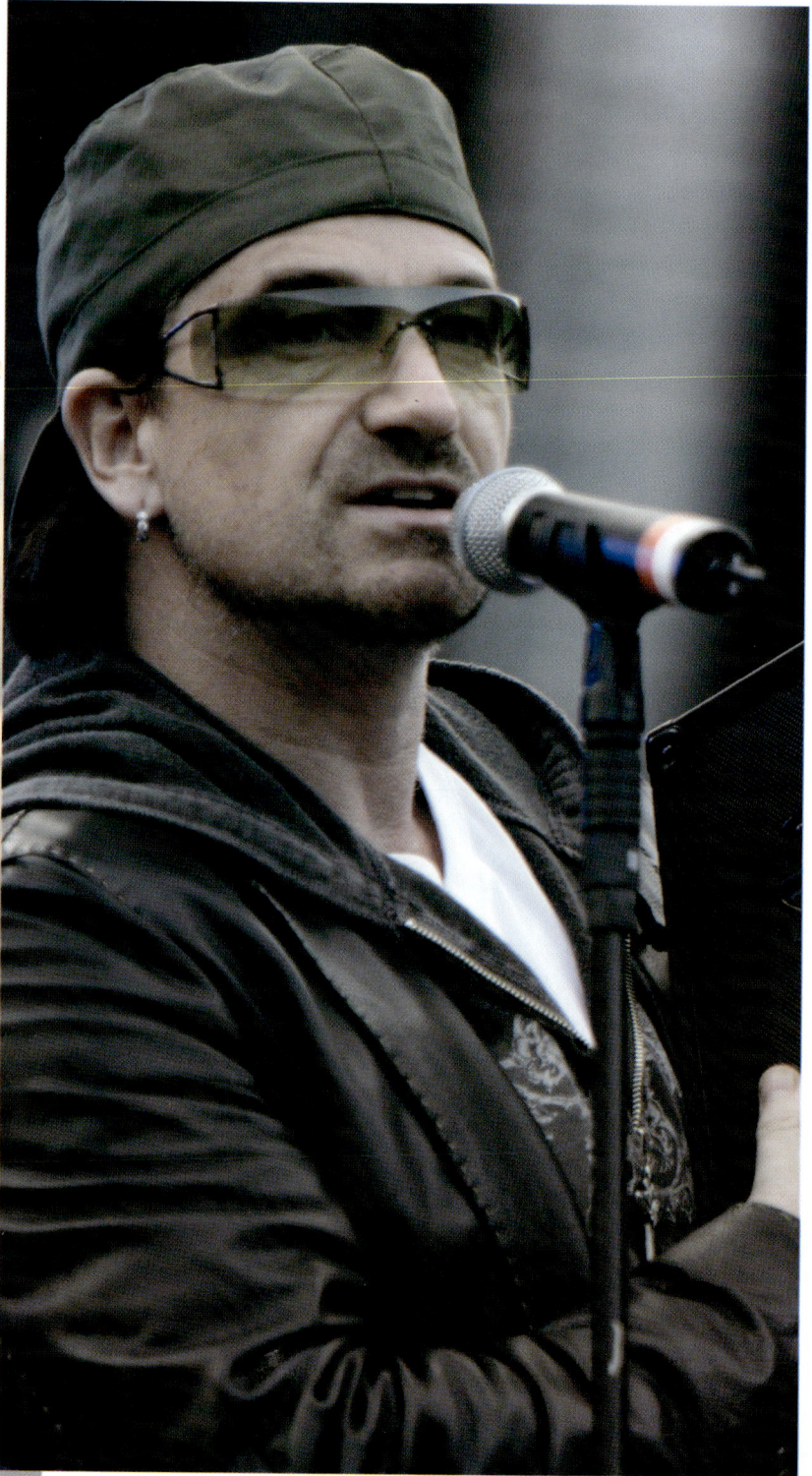

getting involved. One of the stars who's leading the battle is Bono from the rock group U2.

In 1986, World Vision called Bono and asked, "Would you like to see first-hand what's going on in Ethiopia?" In Ethiopia, Bono was confronted with thousands of hungry people—and not enough food to feed them. One man brought his starving child to Bono and said, "If you don't take him, he will surely die." Bono had to refuse, but the experience changed his life. He wrote later, "If the rage rises up inside of me, it's usually him I'm thinking of." That rage has inspired Bono to do all he can to fight poverty and hunger. Today, he is famous around the world, not only because he's a rock star, but also because he's someone who speaks out on behalf of those who need help. And he doesn't just talk. He uses his position to take action.

For instance, Bono was involved in the July 2, 2005 Live 8 concert, an attempt to pressure the G8—leaders of the world's powerful nations—to forgive debts and increase aid for poorer countries. Bono said about the concert, *We are not looking for charity, we are looking for justice.* More than a thousand musicians performed on ten stages around the world, broadcast on almost two hundred stations as millions watched. Almost all the top popular music artists of the world were involved, including the Who, Pink Floyd, Madonna, Mariah Carey, Kanye West, REM, Shakira, Coldplay, Brian Wilson, and U2. Bono and Paul McCartney opened the London show together. Five days after the Live 8 event, world leaders pledged to double aid to Africa from $25 to $50 billion.

NGOs

NGOs—non-governmental organizations—are people who want to change the world who have joined together to form an organization. They're ordinary people who believe so strongly in a particular cause that they get organized, get funding (usually from donations), and get to work. These organizations have become more and more influ-

Did You Know?

The United Nations project to lift African villages out of poverty costs just $110US per person per year for a five-year period. The money comes from governments, partner organizations, and village members—and $50 per person from private donors. This means that your family or your classroom could fund a villager—and do your part to help end poverty and hunger.

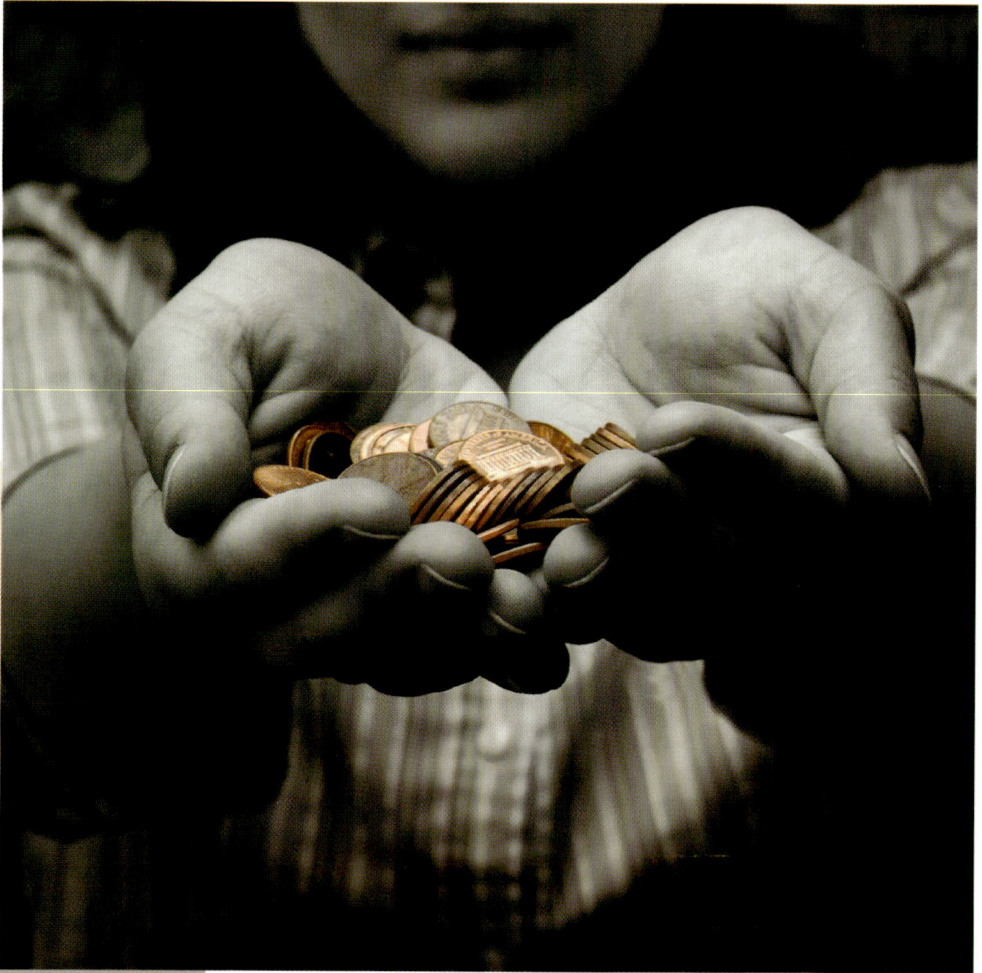

NGOs offer individuals a way to contribute in little ways to big causes.

ential in world affairs. They bring about change socially, economically, and politically.

NGOs get involved with a host of issues, including women's rights, environmental protection, human rights, economic development, political rights, health care—and AIDS and poverty. In many places in the world, NGOs have led the way in spreading democracy, in battling diseases and illnesses, in promoting and enforcing human rights, and in increasing standards of living. Around the world, about 40,000 NGOs operate internationally, but there are even more of these organizations hard at work within various nations; Russia, for example, has 400,000 NGOs, and India has between a million and 2 million! These organizations are working hard to fight both poverty and hunger. The United Nations works with them, and helps them coordinate all their efforts. These organizations prove that individual people can do a lot when they join together.

Author Amartya Sen believes that a shift in attitude is an important part of empowering people to bring about change. He stated:

Hunger and poverty are worldwide problems— that require worldwide, united efforts to solve.

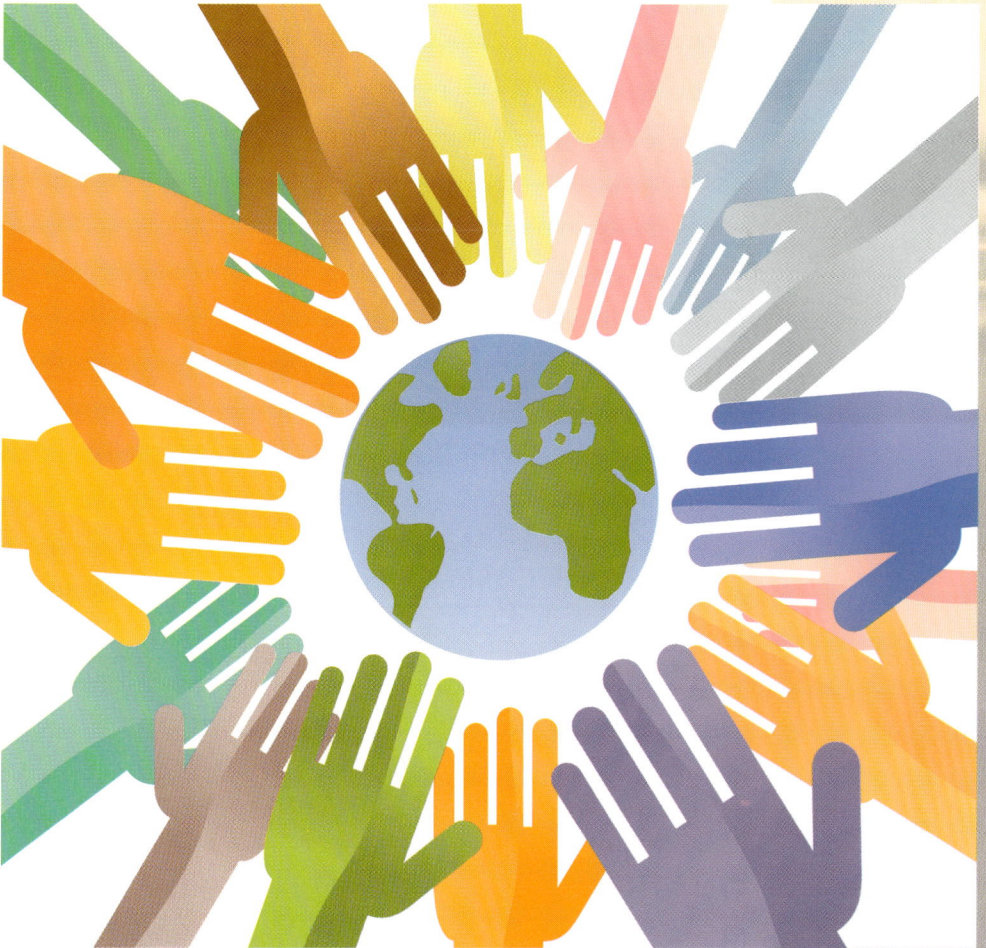

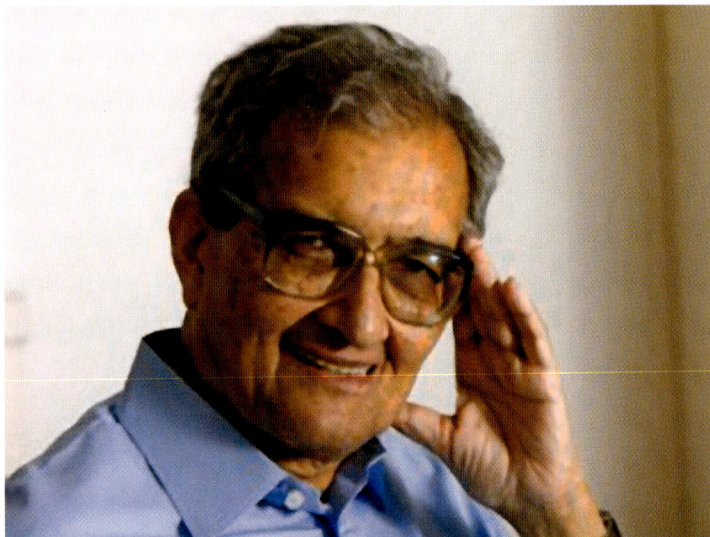

Did You Know?

World Vision is a Christian organization that provides help where people need food, medicine, or shelter; it's one of the charities that's working hard to fight poverty and hunger.

Did You Know?

NGOs became a powerful force in the nineteenth century. They helped end slavery and were the driving force behind women's right to vote.

Public action has to be seen as actions *by* the public and not just as state actions *for* the public. To eliminate the problem of hunger, the political framework of democracy and uncensored press can make a substantial contribution, but it also calls for **activism** of the public. Ultimately, the effectiveness of public action depends not only on legislation, but also on the force and vigour of democratic practice. There is need for moving ahead in different fronts simultaneously to **eradicate** hunger in the modern world. The public is not only the beneficiary of that eradication, but in an important sense, it also has to be its primary instrument. The first step is to see the public as the active agent rather than merely as the long-suffering patient.

Problems as big as hunger and poverty need big solutions. They can only be solved when the entire world—governments, superstars, **grassroots** organizations, and ordinary people like you (the "public" that Sen spoke of)—all work together. The world is depending on each of us.

So let's get started. You never know how much even small efforts can accomplish!

Did You Know?

Because of Bono's charitable work, he was selected by **Time** *magazine as one of the People of the Year for 2005. He is also the only person to have been nominated for an Academy Award, Golden Globe, Grammy, and Nobel Peace Prize. Bono was a nominee for the Nobel Peace Prize in 2003, 2005, and 2006.*

Real People

A person who is making a difference is Dr. Pedro Sanchez. He helped begin the Millennium Villages project, and he leads the science team there. According to the UNAIDS Web site, "The Millennium Villages seek to end extreme poverty by working with the poorest of the poor, village by village throughout Africa, in partnership with governments and other committed stakeholders, providing affordable and science-based solutions to help people lift themselves out of extreme poverty."

Dr. Sanchez's idea meant giving all the villages the things they needed to improve their crops, like better seeds and fertilizers. This first step doubled (and sometimes tripled) the amount of food these villages produced. Now, the project is working to improve farming methods, decreasing dependence on fertilizer and increasing crop diversity. On the Millennium Project Web site, Dr. Sanchez explains, "Crop diversification will do two things: increase the nutritional quality of foods in households and give villagers high value products to sell at the market." In effect, this means the farmers can move from subsistence farming to being small business owners.

What Dr. Sanchez is doing helps achieve the eight Millennium Goals (MDGs). MDG 1—eradicate extreme hunger and poverty—will be tackled, Dr. Sanchez says, because, "Basically, hunger periods are taken care of. For poverty, the transformation will put money in farmers' pockets." Farmers are also providing food for school lunch programs, working to achieve universal primary education (MDG 2). A much greater number of children are now attending school, "because they have a solid meal and are more alert, learn better and play more sports," says Dr. Sanchez. And, schools are attracting many girls who otherwise would not get an education, helping to promote gender equality and empower women (MDG 3). The project also makes women's lives easier, because they will no longer have so many back-breaking chores, such as walking long distances to collect firewood. The project's tree planting adds nitrogen to the soil in the farms, decreasing the need for fertilizer, while it also provides firewood for the villagers. MDGs 4, 5, and 6—reduce child and maternal mortality, and combat HIV/AIDS, malaria, tuberculosis and neglected tropical diseases—are also addressed by Dr. Sanchez's project; he says, "In general, agriculture improves nutrition, and nutrition improves the immune system, making the body more able to combat infections." Ensuring environmental sustainability (MDG 7) is at the core of the kind of agriculture being practiced in the villages, working to increase biodiversity while decreasing erosion and soil run-off. Finally developing a global partnership for development (MDG 8), is the heart of the Millennium Villages project. Dr. Sanchez and the others involved with the project rely on global partners, both public and private, for help.

"I have been personally affected by this project in amazing ways," says Dr. Sanchez. "All my life I have been doing research in experimental plots, but now I find it so exciting to see how people can change—they now have hope. As a professional, it provides evidence that what we have been practicing in science really works. And, as a human being worrying about the bottom billion, to see them pulling themselves out of their poverty traps is very satisfying."

STRAIGHT FROM THE SOURCE

(From Richard H. Roberts, "Readings on Poverty, Hunger, and Economic Development," aculty.plattsburgh.edu/richard. robbins/legacy/hunger_readings.htm)

Food as a Commodity

To understand why people go hungry you must stop thinking about food as something farmers grow for others to eat, and begin thinking about it as something companies produce for other people to buy.

Food is a commodity....

Much of the best agricultural land in the world is used to grow commodities such as cotton, sisal, tea, tobacco, sugar cane, and cocoa, items which are non-food products or are marginally nutritious, but for which there is a large market.

Millions of acres of potentially productive farmland is used to pasture cattle, an extremely inefficient use of land, water and energy, but one for which there is a market in wealthy countries.

More than half the grain grown in the United States (requiring half the water used in the U.S.) is fed to livestock, grain that would feed far more people than would the livestock to which it is fed....

The problem, of course, is that people who don't have enough money to buy food (and more than one billion people earn less than $1.00 a day), simply don't count in the food equation.

In other words, if you don't have the money to buy food, no one is going to grow it for you.

Put yet another way, you would not expect The Gap to manufacture clothes, Adidas to manufacture sneakers, or IBM to provide computers for those people earning $1.00 a day or less; likewise, you would not expect ADM ("Supermarket to the World") to produce food for them.

What this means is that ending hunger requires doing away with poverty, or, at the very least, ensuring that people have enough money or the means to acquire it, to buy, and hence create a market demand for food.

What Do You Think?

- How can people be encouraged to eat more fish?

- How can fish be used to combat food shortages?

- What can people do to get more fish into their diets if they live where fishing has been limited due to water contamination?

Find Out More

Go to these Web sites to find out more about nutrition and your brain:

The Human Brain
222.fi.edu/learn/brain/diet.html

What Is Good Brain Food?
psychologytoday.com/articles/pto-20031028-000010.html

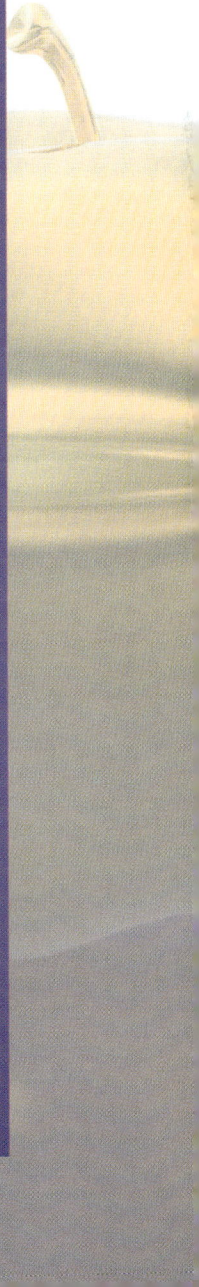

For More Information on Nutrition

Books

Blake, Joan Salge. *Nutrition and You.* San Francisco, Calif.: Benjamin Cummings, 2007.

DK Publishing. *Food.* New York: DK, 2005.

Esherick, Joan. *Diet and Your Emotions: The Comfort Food Falsehood.* Broomall, Pa.: Mason Crest, 2005.

Flynn, Noa. *When Food Is an Enemy: Youth with Eating Disorders.* Broomall, Pa.: Mason Crest, 2008.

Gay, Kathlyn. *Am I Fat? The Obesity Issue for Teens.* Berkeley Heights, N.J.: Enslow, 2006.

Hunnicut, Susan C. *World Hunger.* Farmington Hills, Mich.: Greenhaven, 2006.

Libal, Autumn. *The Importance of Physical Activity and Exercise: The Fitness Factor.* Broomall, Pa.: Mason Crest, 2005.

Nestle, Marion. *Food Politics.* Los Angeles: University of California Press, 2007.

―――. *Safer Food.* Los Angeles: University of California Press, 2004.

Orr, Tamra B. *When the Mirror Lies: Anorexia, Bulimia, and Other Eating Disorders.* New York: Franklin Watts, 2006.

Schlosser, Eric and Charles Wilson. *Chew on This: Everything You Don't Want to Know About Fast Food.* New York: Houghton Mifflin, 2006.

Shanley, Ellen, and Colleen Thompson. *Fueling the Teen Machine*. Palo Alto, Calif.: Bull Publishing, 2001.

Thompson, Janice and Melinda Manore. *Food for Life*. San Francisco, Calif.: Benjamin Cummings, 2006.

Turck, Mary. *Food and Emotions*. Mankato, Minn.: Life-Matters, 2001.

Young, Liz. *World Hunger*. Philadelphia, Pa.: Routledge, 2007.

Web Sites

NRG: Powered by Choice
www.poweredbychoice.org/about/index.php

Nutrition Data
www.nutritiondata.com

Nutrition Explorations
www.nutritionexplorations.org

One
www.one.org

United Nations World Food Program
www.wfp.org/

USDA Food and Nutrition Information Center
fnic.nal.usda.gov/nal_display/index.php?info_center=4&tax_level=1

U.S. Federal Guide to Nutrition
www.nutrition.gov

U.S. My Pyramid
www.mypyramid.gov

World Health Organization
www.who.org

World Hunger: Facts, Figures, and Statistics
library.thinkquest.org/C002291/high/present/stats.htm

World Hunger Notes
www.worldhunger.org/articles/Learn/world%20hunger%
20facts%202002.ht

Glossary of Nutrition-Related Terms

As you read about nutrition and nutrition-related issues, you'll probably come across terms you may not completely understand, even though they may sound familiar. This glossary will help you better understand many of the topics that have to do with nutrition. You may also find it useful for helping you to understand the ingredients listed on food labels.

additives (food additives)
Any natural or synthetic material, other than the basic raw ingredients, in a food item to enhance the final product. Any substance that may affect the characteristics of any food, including those used in the production, processing, treatment, packaging, transportation, or storage of food.

algin
A chemical which comes from algae and is used in puddings, milk shakes, and ice cream to make these foods creamier and thicker and to extend shelf life.

alitame
A sweetener made from amino that offers a taste that is 2000 times sweeter than that of sucrose and can be used in a wide variety of products including beverages, table-top sweeteners, frozen desserts, and baked goods. Since alitame is such an intense sweetener, it is used at very low levels and contributes very few calories. The U.S. FDA is currently considering a petition to approve its use in the United States food supply. So far, alitame has been approved for use in all food and beverage products in Australia, Mexico and New Zealand.

allergen
A food allergen is the part of a food that stimulates the immune system of individuals who are allergic to a specific food. A single food can contain multiple food allergens. Carbohydrates and fats are never allergens, but certain proteins are.

allergy

A food allergy is any adverse reaction to an otherwise harmless food or food component that involves the body's immune system.

alpha carotene

A chemical found in carrots that provides the health benefit of neutralizing free radicals that may cause damage to cells that could lead to cancer.

amino acids

Amino acids function as the building blocks of proteins. They are classified as essential and nonessential and conditionally essential. Essential amino acids cannot be made by the body and must be supplied as part of the diet. Nonessential amino acids can be synthesized by the body in adequate amounts.

anemia

Anemia is a condition in which there are not enough healthy red blood cells, which affects the exchange of oxygen and carbon dioxide between the blood and the body's other cells. Most anemias are caused by a lack of nutrients, but a chronic disease or drugs can cause anemia as well.

anorexia nervosa

An eating disorder that includes weight loss; an intense fear of weight gain or becoming fat, despite the individual's being underweight status; an inaccurate self-awareness body weight or shape; and in females, the absence of at least three consecutive menstrual cycles that would otherwise be expected to occur.

anticarcinogens

Substances that help prevent cancers from forming. More than 600 chemicals are said to be anticancer agents, including natural chemicals in garlic, broccoli, cabbage, and green tea.

antioxidants

Antioxidants may help to maintain overall health. Studies show that antioxidants may be able to help fight off toxic oxygen molecules (often called "free radicals"), a byproduct of metabolism that can damage cells.

ascorbic acid

Also known as vitamin C, it is essential for the development and maintenance of connective tissue. Vitamin C speeds the production of new cells in wound healing and it is an antioxidant that keeps free radicals from hooking up with other molecules to form damaging compounds that might attack tissue. Vitamin C protects the immune system, helps fight off infections, reduces the severity of allergic reactions, and plays a role in the synthesis of hormones and other body chemicals. Green peppers, broccoli, citrus fruits, tomatoes, strawberries, and other fresh fruits and vegetables are good sources of vitamin C.

aspartame

A low calorie sweetener used in a variety of foods and beverages and as a tabletop sweetener. It is about 200 times sweeter than sugar.

beta glucan

A soluble fiber in oats which provides the health benefit of reducing the risk of cardiovascular disease by decreasing circulating blood cholesterol.

BHA

Butylated hydroxyanisole, a chemical compound used to preserve foods by preventing rancidity. BHA is found in foods high in fats and oils; also in meats, cereals, baked goods, beer, and snack foods.

BHT

Butylated hydroxytoluene, a chemical compound used to keep food from changing flavor, odor, and/or color. It is added to foods high in fats and oils and cereals.

BMI
Body Mass Index is an index of a person's weight in relation to height, determined by dividing weight (in kilograms) by the square of the height (in meters).

BMR
Basal Metabolic Rate is the rate of energy used for metabolism when the body is at complete rest.

bulimia nervosa
An eating disorder characterized by rapid consumption of a large amount of food in a short period of time. There are two forms of the condition: purging and non-purging. People with the first type regularly engages in purging through self-induced vomiting or the use of laxatives or diuretics. The non-purging type controls weight through strict dieting, fasting, or excessive exercise.

caffeine
A natural stimulant found in many foods and beverages, including coffee, tea, cola drinks, and chocolate.

calcium
A mineral that you need for strong bones and teeth. Calcium is found in dairy products (like milk and cheese) and also in dried beans and dark green vegetables (like spinach).

calorie
A unit of measure, sometimes referred to as a kilocalorie. Calories measure the amount of energy your body can get from a food. Calories are found in fats, carbohydrates, proteins, and alcohol.

carbohydrates
Sugars and starches are the main forms of carbohydrates. Sugars are simple carbohydrates and starches, such as breads, cereals and pasta, are complex carbohydrates. Each gram of carbohydrate provides 4 calories of energy.

carcinogens
Substances that cause cancer within the body.

carotene
Also known as beta-carotene, a yellow pigment (found in food) that may be converted into Vitamin A in the body.

catechins
A chemical found in tea which provides the health benefits of neutralizing free radicals and possibly reducing the risk of cancer.

cholesterol
Cholesterol is a soft, waxy substance found among the lipids (fats) in the bloodstream and in all your body's cells. It is used to form cell membranes, some hormones and other needed tissues. However, a high level of cholesterol in the blood is a major risk factor for coronary heart disease.

coronary heart disease
Conditions related to the heart and blood vessels leading to and from the heart. Most common symptoms are chest pains, heart attacks, stroke, and high blood pressure.

cyclamate
A sweetener that is 30 times sweeter than sucrose and calorie free. It is approved for tabletop use in Canada and more than 50 countries in Europe, Asia, South America and Africa. Since 1970, however, the use of cyclamate has been banned in the United States on the basis of a study that suggested that cyclamates may be related to the development of bladder tumors in rats.

diabetes
A group of medical disorders characterized by high blood sugar levels. Normally when people eat, food is digested and much of it is converted to glucose—a simple sugar— which the body uses for energy. The blood carries the glu-

cose to cells where it is absorbed with the help of the hormone insulin. For people with diabetes, however, the body does not make enough insulin, or cannot properly use the insulin it does make. Without insulin, glucose accumulates in the blood rather than moving into the cells. High blood sugar levels result.

diet
What you eat every day.

digestion
The process where your body breaks down food into smaller parts it can use.

eating disorders
Psychological conditions where a person's relationship with food becomes unhealthy. Bulimia and anorexia are both examples.

energy
The body's capacity for doing work. Food gives us the energy we need to live, work, and play.

enriched
Indicates that more of the food's natural nutrients have been added during processing. This is often done to replace nutrients that may have been lost through handling.

fat
These are concentrated sources of energy. Every gram of fat provides 9 calories.

fat replacers
Fat replacers are developed to duplicate the taste and texture of fat, but contain fewer calories per gram than fat.

fiber
Part of plants which the body cannot digest, it helps your digestive system and intestines keep working well.

5 A Day
The dietary recommendation to consume five servings of fruits and vegetables every day.

flavanones
A chemical found in citrus fruits that provides the health benefits of neutralizing **free radicals** and possibly reducing the risk of cancer.

flavones
A chemical found in various fruits and vegetables that provides the health benefits of neutralizing **free radicals** and possibly reducing the risk of cancer.

folic acid
Chemicals that help with the digestion of protein. Good dietary sources of folate include leafy, dark green vegetables, legumes, citrus fruits and juices, peanuts, whole grains, and fortified breakfast cereals. Recent studies show that if all women of childbearing age consumed sufficient folic acid (either through diet or supplements), 50 to 70 percent of birth defects of the brain and spinal cord could be prevented.

food intolerance
A general term for any adverse reaction to a food or food component that does not involve the body's immune system.

food preservatives
Preservatives prevent spoilage either by slowing the growth of organisms that live on food or by protecting the food from oxygen.

fortified
When that nutrients not naturally found in that particular food have been added during processing to enhance nutrition.

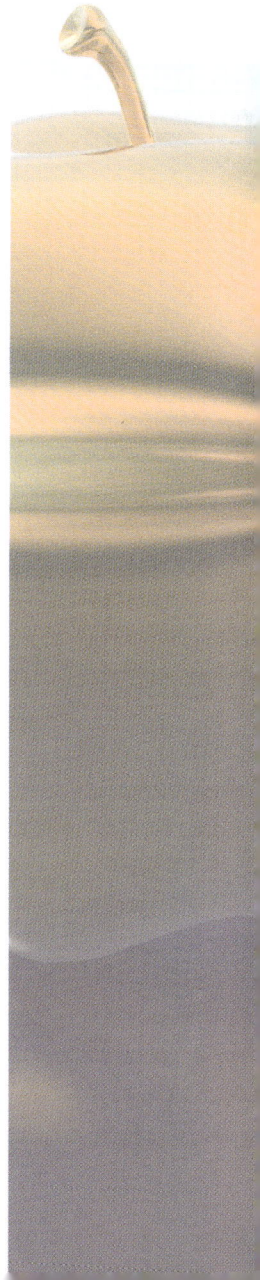

free radicals
Chemicals released when unsaturated fatty acids decompose and which may contribute to cancer growth.

fructose
Fructose is a sugar found naturally in fruits; it is also a component of high fructose corn syrup.

glucose
A natural sugar that comes from grape juice, honey, and certain vegetables, among other things.

glycerin
A syrupy type of alcohol derived from sugar that is used in food flavorings to maintain desired food consistency.

glycerol
A colorless, odorless, syrupy liquid that is obtained from fats and oils and used to retain moisture and add sweetness to foods.

grains
The seeds or fruits of various food plants, including cereal grasses, such as wheat, corn, oats, barley, rye, and rice. Grain foods include foods such as bread, cereals, rice, and pasta.

guar gum
A substance made from the seeds of the guar plant that acts as a stabilizer in foods. Is found as a food additive in cheese, ice cream, and dressings.

high fructose corn syrup
A sweet syrup that generally contains 42 percent, 55 percent or 90 percent fructose, which is used in products such as soft drinks or cake mixes.

iron
A mineral that is an important part of hemoglobin, your blood's oxygen-carrying molecule within red blood cells.

Iron also helps your body resist infection and use energy from food.

lactose intolerance
Lactose intolerance is an inherited inability to properly digest dairy products. Symptoms of lactose intolerance, including abdominal cramps, gas, and diarrhea, can increase with age.

lecithin
A byproduct of soybean oil, it is also found in eggs, red meats, spinach, and nuts. It is used in some commercial foods as a lubricant, and it promotes "good" cholesterol levels.

lipids
Chemicals that include fats and oils.

lycopene
The chemical that gives tomatoes and some other fruits and vegetables their red color. It is a good antioxidant that helps keep cells healthy.

malnutrition
Poor nutrition resulting in tiredness, illness, lack of ability to fight infection, and finally muscle wasting in the latter stages.

metabolism
The chemical reactions that go on in living cells by which energy is produced for use by the cells.

MSG (monosodium glutamate)
A flavoring found in many packaged foods and in Chinese foods. In the early part of the century, MSG was extracted from seaweed and other plant sources. Today, MSG is produced in many countries around the world through a fermentation process of molasses from sugar cane or sugar beets, as well as starch and corn sugar.

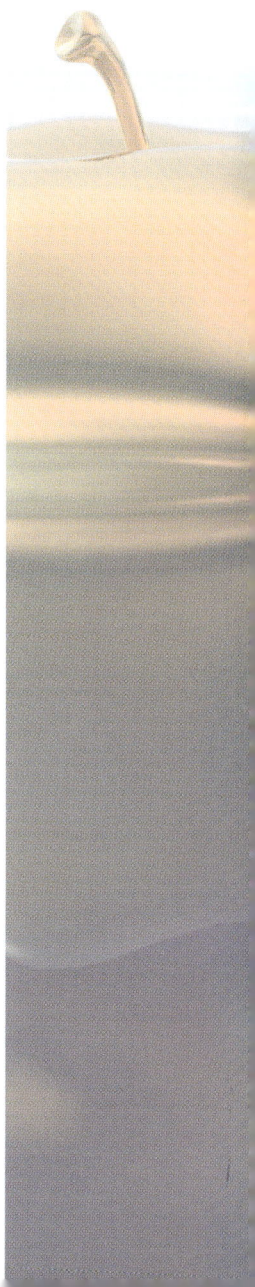

nitrite
Nitrite is a food additive that has been used for centuries to preserve meats, fish and poultry. It also contributes to the characteristic flavor, color, and texture of processed meats such as hot dogs.

nutrients
Components in food that our bodies use for survival, including fats, carbohydrates, protein, vitamins, and minerals.

nutrient density
Nutrient-dense foods are those that provide substantial amounts of vitamins and minerals and relatively fewer calories. The opposite of nutrient dense is calorie dense, foods that mainly supply calories and relatively few nutrients.

obesity
A chronic disease characterized by excessively high body fat in relation to lean body tissue.

omega 3 fatty acids
A type of fatty acid found in fish and marine oils that provide the health benefits of reduced risk of cardiovascular disease and improved mental and visual function.

organic
Agricultural products that are grown using cultural, biological, and mechanical methods rather than chemicals to control pests, improve soil quality, and enhance processing.

overweight
An excess of body fat.

phytochemicals
Chemicals found in plants and vegetables, some of which have been found to help protect against some cancers, heart disease, and other chronic health conditions.

poultry
Meat that comes from birds, like chickens, ducks, geese, and turkeys.

protein
Building blocks that our body uses, which are made up of chains of amino acids. Body tissues, like our skin, hair, and muscles, are built mostly of protein. Protein is also needed for our bodies' growth and repair.

refined
Refers to the fine grinding and sifting of cereal grains to produce white flour.

saccharin
Saccharin is the oldest of the "artificial" sweeteners. It is 300 times sweeter than sucrose, heat stable, and does not promote dental cavities. Saccharin has a long shelf life, but a slightly bitter aftertaste. It is not metabolized in the human digestive system, is excreted rapidly in the urine, and does not accumulate in body.

saturated fat
Fatty acids that have all the hydrogen they can hold on their chemical chains. They mainly come from animal foods and tend to deposit in blood vessels, blocking blood flow.

sodium (Na)
Part of the chemical that makes up table salt. This mineral is used for cellular fluid balance and muscle retractions.

sodium nitrite
A salt used in smoked or cured fish and in meat curing preparation. It acts as a preservative and color fixative. Can combine with chemicals in the stomach to form a carcinogenic substance.

soluble fiber
A type of dietary fiber found in psyllium, cereals, oatmeal, apples, citrus fruits, beans, and other foods that reduce

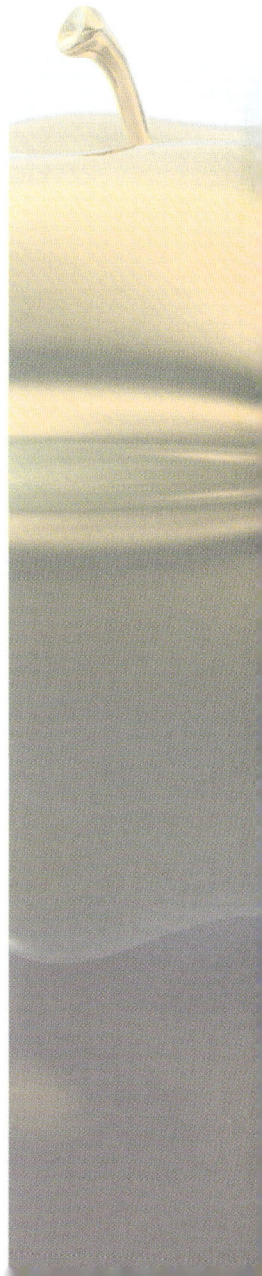

high blood cholesterol levels, which in turn decreases the risk of cardiovascular disease.

soy protein
The protein found in soybeans and soy-based foods, which when consumed at the level of 25 grams per day may reduce the risk of heart disease.

starch
A complex carbohydrate that our bodies breaks down and uses for energy.

sugar
A simple carbohydrate that our bodies breaks down and uses for energy.

sulfites
Sulfiting agents are sometimes used to preserve the color of foods such as dried fruits and vegetable, and to inhibit the growth of microorganisms in fermented foods such as wine. Sulfites are safe for most people. A small segment of the population, however, has been found to develop shortness of breath or fatal shock shortly after exposure to these preservatives. Sulfites can provoke severe asthma attacks in sulfite sensitive asthmatics. For that reason, in 1986 the U.S. FDA banned the use of sulfites on fresh fruits and vegetables (except potatoes) intended to be sold or served raw to consumers. Sulfites added to all packaged and processed foods must be listed on the product label.

trans fats
Trans fats occur naturally in many meats, butter, and milk, as well as in commercially prepared margarines and solid cooking fats. The main sources of trans fats in people's diet today are margarine, shortening, commercial frying fats, and high-fat baked goods. Trans fats can raise "bad" cholesterol and lower "good" cholesterol.

triglycerides
The scientific name for the common form of fat, found in both the body and in foods. Most body fat is stored in the form of triglycerides.

unsaturated fat
This type of fat has been found to be better for health and may protect against heart disease. It is mainly found in vegetables and fish.

vegetarian
A person whose diet excludes some or all protein from animal sources. Semi-vegetarians will not eat red meat but will eat fish and poultry. Lacto-ovo vegetarians eat no meats but will eat dairy products and eggs. Lacto vegetarians eat no meat, only dairy products. Vegans are strict vegetarians, and eat no foods from animals at all, only from plant sources.

vitamins
A group of nutrients that our bodies need to grow and function well. Some important vitamins that we need are B vitamins, and vitamin A, C, D, E and K.

whole grain
A term that applies to grains in which the outer layer, where the B vitamins and minerals are concentrated, is not removed during processing.

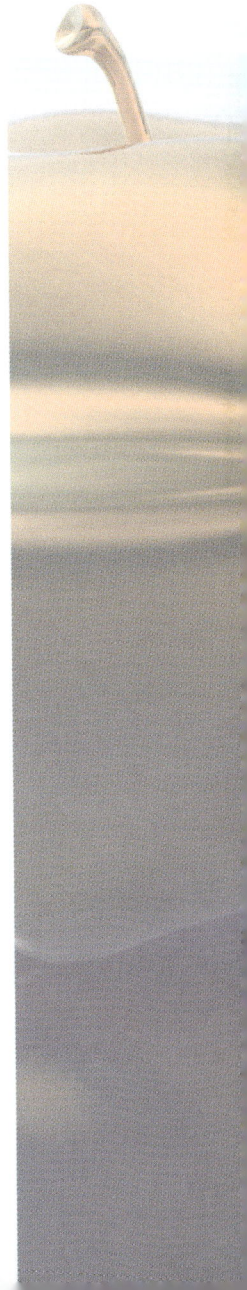

Bibliography

ACC/SCN (United Nations Administrative Committee on Coordination/Sub-Committee on Nutrition). Fourth Report on the World Nutrition Situation. Geneva: ACC/SCN in collaboration with IFPRI, 2000.

Asfaw, Abay. "Obesity and Chronic Diseases: Not Limited to the Affluent." International Food Policy Research Institute. http://www.ifpri.org/pubs/newsletters/IFPRI-Forum/200612/if17

Behrman, J., and M. Rosenzweig. The Returns to Increasing Body Weight. Philadelphia, Penn.: Department of Economics, University of Pennsylvania, 2001.

Britten, Patricia, Kristin Marcoe, Sedigheh Yamini, and Carole Davis. "Development of Food Intake Patterns for the MyPyramid Food Guidance System." J. Nutrition Education and Behavior vol. 38 (December 2006): S78–S92.

Che, J. and J. Chen. "Food insecurity in Canadian Households." Health Reports (Statistics Canada, catalogue 82-003). 2001;12:11–22.

Damsgaard, C. T., L. Lauritzen, and T. M. Kjaer. "Fish Oil Supplementation Modulates Immune Function in Healthy Infants." J. Nutrition vol. 137 (April 2007): 1031–1036.

"Diet and Nutrition." Time. http://www.time.com/time/archive/collections/0,21428,c_diet_and_nutrition,00.shtml.

"Eat the Basic 7 Every Day." http://digital.library.unt.edu/permalink/meta-dc-619:1.

Farney, Teresa J. "Good Mood Food: Researchers Find Links Between Nutrition and the Brain Chemicals Governing Our Inner World." The Gazette, September 18, 2002.

Food Research and Action Center. "Hunger and Obesity? Making the Connection." www.frac.org/pdf/Paradox.pdf

———. "The Impact of Rising Food Costs on Low-Income Americans." April 17, 2008. www.frac.org/pdf/factsheet_foodcosts_apr08.pdf

Gardner, G., and B. Halweil. Underfed and Overfed: The Global Epidemic of Malnutrition. Worldwatch Paper 150. Washington, D.C.: Worldwatch Institute, 2000.

Gillespie, S., and L. Haddad. Attacking the Double Burden of Malnutrition in Asia and the Pacific. Policy Paper. Manila: Asian Development Bank, 2001.

Green, K. N., H. Martinez-Coria, and H. Khashwji. "Dietary docosahexaenoic acid and docosapentaenoic acid ameliorate amyloid-beta and tau pathology via a mechanism involving presenilin 1 levels." J. Neuroscience vol. 27 (April 2007): 4385–4395.

Hoddinott, J., M. Adato, T. Besley, and L. Haddad. Participation and Poverty Reduction: Issues, Theory, and New Evidence from South Africa. Food Consumption and Nutrition Division Discussion Paper 98. Washington, D.C.: International Food Policy Research Institute, 2001.

International Food Information Council. "Child & Adolescent Nutrition, Health & Physical Activity." http://ific.org/nutrition/kids/index.cfm?renderforprint=1.

Maluccio,J.,L.Haddad,and J.May. 2000. Social capital and welfare in South Africa,1993-1998.Journal of Development Studies 36 (6): 54–81.

Minister of Public Works and Government Services Canada. Nutrition and Healthy Aging: Workshop on health aging. 2002. www.phac-aspc.gc.ca/seniors-aines/pubs/workshop_healthyaging/nutrition/nutrition1_e.htm.

Popkin,B. M., S. Horton, and S. Kim. The Nutrition Transition and Diet-Related Chronic Diseases in Asia: Implications for Prevention. Chapel Hill, N.C.: Department of Nutrition and Carolina Population Center, 2001.

Sen, Amartya. "Public Action to Remedy Hunger." The Hunger Project. www.thp.org/reports/sen/sen890.htm

Squires, Sally. "Pyramid Schemes: Taking a Global Perspective on Nutrition."Washington Post, July 4, 2000.

Stang, J., and M. Story (eds.). Guidelines for Adolescent Nutrition Services. Minneapolis: University of Minnesota, 2005.

Valentine, Vicky. "The Causes Behind Hunger in America."Hunger in America. NPR. November 22, 2005, www.npr.org/templates/story/story.php?storyId=5021812

WHO. FAO/WHO Launch Expert Report on Diet, Nutrition, and Prevention of Chronic Diseases." 2003. http://www.who.int/mediacentre/news/releases/2003/pr32/en.

Willett, Walter C., and P. J. Skettett. Eat, Drink, and Be Healthy: The Harvard Medical School Guide to Healthy Eating. New York: Free Press, 2005.

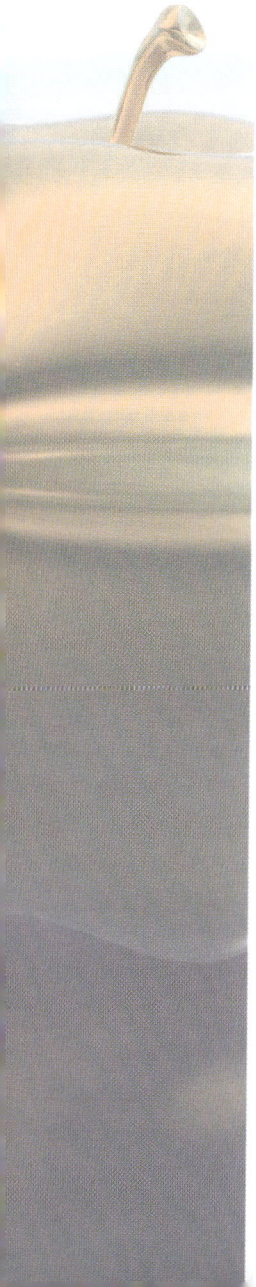

Wolfe, WS, E.A. Frongillo, and P. Valois "Understanding the Experience of Food Insecurity by Elders Suggests Ways to Improve Its Measurement." The Journal of Nutrition 2003;133:2762–69.

Index

Africa 31–32, 34–36, 44, 47, 56, 76, 81, 86
amino acids 13, 20
Annan, Kofi 78
Australia 22

Bono 74, 80–81, 85
brain 10, 20, 89

calcium 16, 19, 50
calorie 8, 10–16, 20, 47, 66, 67, 69
Canada 22–23
carbohydrates 8–13, 20–22, 47
Chad 56
chemicals 14, 18
children 10–11, 20, 22, 24–26, 30, 32, 35, 37, 39–40, 42–43, 46–49, 62, 64, 66, 69, 77–78, 86
crime 69

deficiency 9, 11, 22, 24, 46
democratic 57, 84
developed country 9, 11–12, 14, 18, 20, 22, 25, 27, 31, 37–38, 46, 50, 52, 59, 60, 62, 64, 66, 78
developing country 9, 12–13, 19–20, 34, 39, 42, 44–47, 49–53, 55, 57, 59, 62, 66, 71, 71, 87
diet 10–12, 14, 19, 21–22, 25, 47, 49, 64, 66, 73, 89
disease 6, 10, 14, 15, 18, 34, 42, 62, 78, 87,
distribution 50, 59
drought 39, 44, 53

Earth 20, 34, 41, 54, 57

economics 6, 7, 9, 34, 37, 54, 56, 58, 60–61, 70, 74, 82, 84, 88
environment 28, 39, 42, 44, 52, 78, 82, 87
Ethiopia 56, 81
European Union 32

famine 44, 53–53, 56–57, 59
farmland 39, 47, 50
fat 8, 10, 11, 13–16, 19–23, 33, 47, 66–68, 70
fiber 8–11, 13–14,
fish 13, 15, 21, 53, 89
food insecurity 37, 60, 70

G8 81
global 28, 31, 42, 78
gram 8, 10, 12, 16, 50, 70, 85–86
Great Britain 22

health care 28, 31–32, 38–39, 40–42, 70, 82
hormones 14
human rights 44, 53, 57, 71, 82

iodine 20, 24, 46, 50, 62
India 22, 32, 38, 44, 47–48, 50, 73, 83
injustice 77
iron 18, 20, 22, 24–25, 28, 39, 42, 44, 52, 62, 78, 82

Japan 25
job 8, 32–33, 39, 41, 68, 70, 79

label 10–11, 15,
Latin America 36, 47
latino 62

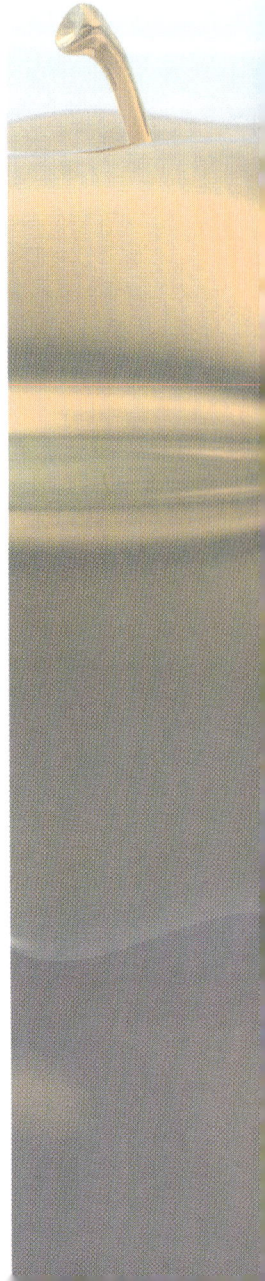

legumes 13
Live 8 81

malnutrition 10, 22, 40, 44, 48–50, 57, 60, 62, 66, 71, 74, 77
McHugh, Kathleen 32
micronutrients 11
military 56–57
Millennium Project, The 59, 74, 77–79, 86–87
minerals 8–11, 18–19, 49, 67
mortality 60, 62, 64, 77, 87

nervous system 10, 14
Nigeria 56
Non-Governmental Organizations(NGOs) 7, 34, 56, 74, 79, 81–84
nutrients 8, 10–11, 20, 42, 47, 49, 66–67

obesity 11, 14, 20, 60, 64, 66–68, 70

pregnant 10, 22, 62, 64, 66
protein 8, 10–13, 15–16, 18–21, 23, 47, 49, 62, 67,
pyramid, food 20, 21, 27

Russia 83

Sen, Amartya 56, 84
sodium 19
Somalia 56
sports 69, 87
starvation 46, 49, 58
stress 70
Sudan 31, 36, 56
sugar 11, 13, 20, 22, 50, 88,

trade 56, 70, 78

U2 74, 81
undernourishment 62, 66, 71
Uganda 56
United Nations 7, 30, 41, 64, 71, 74, 77–79, 83
United States 20, 22, 31, 37–38, 43, 48, 62, 64, 88
United States Department of Agriculture 27, 62

Picture Credits

Dreamstime
  AbsolutPhotos: p. 28–29   Tiero: p. 35
  Aprescinder: p. 30   TravelingLight: p. 66
  Bernardo66: 44–45
  Fleyeing: p. 33   Health Canada
  Jahoo: p. 10   p. 23
  Jgroup: p. 74–75
  JojoBob: p. 69   iStockphoto
  Mattphoto: p. 36   pp. 76, 79, 82–83
  PureRadianceJennifer:
  60–61   Jupiter Images
  Racnus: p. 52   pp. 9, 12, 14, 17, 19, 64
  RCHPhotos: p. 51
  StuartKey: p. 63   USDA
  TheFinalMiracle: p. 38,   p. 21
  48–49

To the best knowledge of the publisher, all other images are in the
public domain. If any image has been inadvertently uncredited,
please notify Harding House Publishing Service, Vestal, New York
13850, so that rectification can be made for future printings.

About the Author

Rae Simons is the author of many books for children and young adults. She lives in upstate New York with her family.

About the Consultant

Elise DeVore Berlan, MD, MPH, FAAP, is a faculty member of the Division of Adolescent Health at Nationwide Children's Hospital and an Assistant Professor of Clinical Pediatrics at The Ohio State University College of Medicine. She completed her Fellowship in Adolescent Medicine at Children's Hospital Boston and obtained a Master's Degree in Public Health at the Harvard School of Public Health. Dr. Berlan completed her residency in pediatrics at the Children's Hospital of Philadelphia, where she also served an additional year as Chief Resident. She received her medical degree from the University of Iowa College of Medicine. Dr. Berlan is board certified in Pediatrics and board eligible in Adolescent Medicine. She provides primary care and consultative services in the area of Young Women's Health, including gynecological problems, concerns about puberty, reproductive health services, and reproductive endocrine disorders.

Peter Vash, M.D., is a Professor of Medicine at UCLA Medical Center. He is a Fellow of the American Association of Clinical Endocrinologists and a board-certified internist specializing in metabolism and obesity. He is also the author of *The Fat to Muscle Diet*, *The Dieter's Dictionary*, and *A Matter of Fat*.

poultry
Meat that comes from birds, like chickens, ducks, geese, and turkeys.

protein
Building blocks that our body uses, which are made up of chains of amino acids. Body tissues, like our skin, hair, and muscles, are built mostly of protein. Protein is also needed for our bodies' growth and repair.

refined
Refers to the fine grinding and sifting of cereal grains to produce white flour.

saccharin
Saccharin is the oldest of the "artificial" sweeteners. It is 300 times sweeter than sucrose, heat stable, and does not promote dental cavities. Saccharin has a long shelf life, but a slightly bitter aftertaste. It is not metabolized in the human digestive system, is excreted rapidly in the urine, and does not accumulate in body.

saturated fat
Fatty acids that have all the hydrogen they can hold on their chemical chains. They mainly come from animal foods and tend to deposit in blood vessels, blocking blood flow.

sodium (Na)
Part of the chemical that makes up table salt. This mineral is used for cellular fluid balance and muscle retractions.

sodium nitrite
A salt used in smoked or cured fish and in meat curing preparation. It acts as a preservative and color fixative. Can combine with chemicals in the stomach to form a carcinogenic substance.

soluble fiber
A type of dietary fiber found in psyllium, cereals, oatmeal, apples, citrus fruits, beans, and other foods that reduce

high blood cholesterol levels, which in turn decreases the risk of cardiovascular disease.

soy protein
The protein found in soybeans and soy-based foods, which when consumed at the level of 25 grams per day may reduce the risk of heart disease.

starch
A complex carbohydrate that our bodies breaks down and uses for energy.

sugar
A simple carbohydrate that our bodies breaks down and uses for energy.

sulfites
Sulfiting agents are sometimes used to preserve the color of foods such as dried fruits and vegetable, and to inhibit the growth of microorganisms in fermented foods such as wine. Sulfites are safe for most people. A small segment of the population, however, has been found to develop shortness of breath or fatal shock shortly after exposure to these preservatives. Sulfites can provoke severe asthma attacks in sulfite sensitive asthmatics. For that reason, in 1986 the U.S. FDA banned the use of sulfites on fresh fruits and vegetables (except potatoes) intended to be sold or served raw to consumers. Sulfites added to all packaged and processed foods must be listed on the product label.

trans fats
Trans fats occur naturally in many meats, butter, and milk, as well as in commercially prepared margarines and solid cooking fats. The main sources of trans fats in people's diet today are margarine, shortening, commercial frying fats, and high-fat baked goods. Trans fats can raise "bad" cholesterol and lower "good" cholesterol.

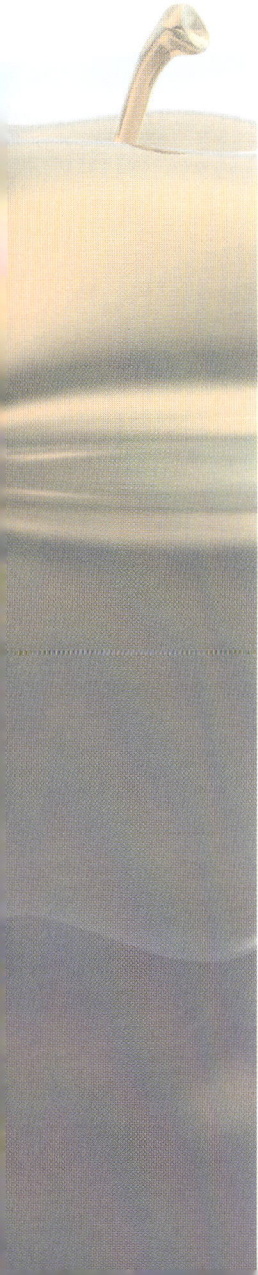

triglycerides
The scientific name for the common form of fat, found in both the body and in foods. Most body fat is stored in the form of triglycerides.

unsaturated fat
This type of fat has been found to be better for health and may protect against heart disease. It is mainly found in vegetables and fish.

vegetarian
A person whose diet excludes some or all protein from animal sources. Semi-vegetarians will not eat red meat but will eat fish and poultry. Lacto-ovo vegetarians eat no meats but will eat dairy products and eggs. Lacto vegetarians eat no meat, only dairy products. Vegans are strict vegetarians, and eat no foods from animals at all, only from plant sources.

vitamins
A group of nutrients that our bodies need to grow and function well. Some important vitamins that we need are B vitamins, and vitamin A, C, D, E and K.

whole grain
A term that applies to grains in which the outer layer, where the B vitamins and minerals are concentrated, is not removed during processing.

Bibliography

ACC/SCN (United Nations Administrative Committee on Coordination/Sub-Committee on Nutrition). Fourth Report on the World Nutrition Situation. Geneva: ACC/SCN in collaboration with IFPRI, 2000.

Asfaw, Abay. "Obesity and Chronic Diseases: Not Limited to the Affluent." International Food Policy Research Institute. http://www.ifpri.org/pubs/newsletters/IFPRI-Forum/200612/if17

Behrman, J., and M. Rosenzweig. The Returns to Increasing Body Weight. Philadelphia, Penn.: Department of Economics, University of Pennsylvania, 2001.

Britten, Patricia, Kristin Marcoe, Sedigheh Yamini, and Carole Davis. "Development of Food Intake Patterns for the MyPyramid Food Guidance System." J. Nutrition Education and Behavior vol. 38 (December 2006): S78–S92.

Che, J. and J. Chen. "Food insecurity in Canadian Households." Health Reports (Statistics Canada, catalogue 82-003). 2001;12:11–22.

Damsgaard, C. T., L. Lauritzen, and T. M. Kjaer. "Fish Oil Supplementation Modulates Immune Function in Healthy Infants." J. Nutrition vol. 137 (April 2007): 1031–1036.

"Diet and Nutrition." Time. http://www.time.com/time/archive/collections/0,21428,c_diet_and_nutrition,00.shtml.

"Eat the Basic 7 Every Day." http://digital.library.unt.edu/permalink/meta-dc-619:1.